Marisa Peer studied hypno............ing
Institute of Los Angeles, kn............ning
institute in the world, she ;............1 of
nutrition. She has spent over twenty years working ....isive
client list including royalty, rock stars, actors, professional and
Olympic athletes, CEOs and media personalities and has developed
her own unique style that is frequently referred to as life-changing.
Marisa works extensively on television and radio, including her
appearance on *Celebrity Fit Club* UK and USA, was named the
Best British Therapist by *Men's Health* magazine in May 2006 and
featured in *Tatler*'s 2007 Guide to Britain's 250 Best Doctors. She
gives lectures and workshops all over the world. Marisa's latest
book *Ultimate Confidence* is now available from Sphere. Visit her
website at *www.marisapeer.com*.

Praise for Marisa Peer

I would recommend this book to my patients or anyone who wishes
to change their weight and find a healthy relationship with food.
Marisa Peer is caring rather than critical and understands the
complex issues involved in weight loss. Marisa works on the premise
that dieting alone does not work long term for the majority of
overweight people. Instead, if we change our mindset not only is it
easier to become slimmer it is easier to remain that way. *You Can Be
Thin* shows the reader how to achieve this change and is very
different to other diet books as Marisa has a very different and
unique approach that works.
Dr Chris Steele MB ChB
GP and resident doctor on ITV's *This Morning*
Health Journalist of the Year 2007

In *You Can Be Thin* Marisa Peer offers an insightful, entertaining and caring psychological approach to weight loss and management. Achieving and sustaining weight loss involves understanding your relationship with food and knowing how to change it for good. Marisa shows the reader how to do this and how to make it last. This book will guide you to the body you always dreamed of.

Dr Adam Carey BSc MBBChir DFFP MRC Fel, MRCOG CST
Leading nutritionist and nutritional adviser to the England Rugby and England Cricket teams

You Can Be Thin provides refreshing inspiration to achieve a healthy lifestyle in a simple and logical way and is in complete harmony with current medical thinking. The most important message, as always, is to define an improved quality of life for oneself. In this book Marisa's approach, combined with her personality and humour, works with the reader to make this possible.

Dr Susan Horsewood-Lee MB BS MRCGP
Renowned British General Practitioner

YOU CAN BE THIN

The Ultimate Hypnosis Programme
to End Dieting ... Forever

MARISA PEER

SPHERE

First published in Great Britain in 2008 by Sphere
This edition published in 2015 by Sphere

10 9 8 7 6

Copyright © Marisa Peer 2008

The moral right of the author has been asserted.

A CIP catalogue record for this book
is available from the British Library.

ISBN 978-0-7515-4295-0

Typeset in Sabon by M Rules
Printed and bound in Great Britain by
Clays Ltd, Elcograf S.p.A.

Papers used by Sphere are from well-managed forests
and other responsible sources.

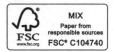

Sphere
An imprint of
Little, Brown Book Group
Carmelite House
50 Victoria Embankment
London EC4Y 0DZ

An Hachette UK Company
www.hachette.co.uk

www.littlebrown.co.uk

Contents

To download the free hypnosis sessions which accompany the book please go to:
www.marisapeer.com/youcanbethindownload
Password: marisa

This book is dedicated to the memory of the very brave and very beautiful Sasha Jeffrey.

Very special thanks and acknowledgements to my amazing friends, especially Claudia Rosencrantz, who made all this possible, Daniela Neumann, Helen Barbour, Jessica Richards, Maria and Gordon Thomson and Charles Montagu for pushing me to do my seminars, for reading my manuscripts and always believing in me and this book. I could not ask for better friends. If ever there were a design for the perfect friend you would be the template.

To my mother Dee Saddler and father Ronald Peer and all my family, especially my very special and lovely Phaedra. To Isaac, Bree and Lucas for always making me laugh. To Cissie for everything.

To Dagmar Charlton for putting me on television in America and giving me the best experience and such happy memories.

A huge thank you to Dr Susan Horsewood Lee, Dr Adam Carey and Dr Chris Steele for being so supportive of the work I do.

To Sarah Rustin for being a fabulous editor and to Eugenie Furniss, my amazing agent. To Kirsteen Astor for great publicity, and everyone at Little, Brown for being extraordinary. Thanks also to my own wonderful teachers Gil Boyne, Wayne Dyer, Brian Tracey, David Viscott, Tony Robbins: all such giving people who taught me so much.

To my lovely husband John, for your love and patience.

And finally to all my clients over the years, you have taught me as much as I ever taught you, thank you.

Why This Works But Diets Don't

Every diet asks you to change, it asks you to change your eating habits until you have lost some weight or reached your ideal weight and then the rest is up to you. I am going to show you how to change things other than the amount you eat in ways that will work, so you won't feel cast adrift as you do when diets fail. Throughout this book I will focus on the methods that really achieve a lasting effect on your body. You are going to change your attitude, your language, your thinking, your whole mindset to reach your ideal weight and stay that way for good. *You Can Be Thin* is written in a very specific hypnotic style that is designed to help you re-evaluate and re-address your entire relationship with food and your body. Just reading this book and interacting with the exercises within it will give you not only a crucial understanding of why you do what you do, it will also show you how to change forever in a way that is powerful and liberating.

The beauty of this book is that the repetition within it is designed to do all the work for you as you absorb the instructions and become fully receptive to change. This book is an amazing programme because it is not just about how you eat and your attitude to food, it is about your whole outlook on life. That is why it is so worth your time to read it and do the exercises. You might just find it's the best investment you ever made. The hypnotic commands in this book don't require you to do what I say; it's not about rigidly following my advice or rules. Instead, the hypnosis triggers you to review what I say, absorb the information and then naturally implement changes, changes that are amazingly effective. By the end of this book you will have changed your entire relationship with food for the better and forever and you will enjoy the whole process, so get ready to make great changes to your body and sustain the change.

The method behind *You Can Be Thin* is unique in that it covers everything that causes overeating as well as providing the answers that offer a lifelong cure without having to diet. In addition to the hypnosis that will end the cravings for foods that cause weight gain, the programme's steps include tests to take that identify exactly what type of eater you are followed by an effective cure for each type, as well as corresponding case histories to relate to and learn from. It includes proven habit breakers and proven psychological techniques that get results and free you from overeating and being overweight, as well as accurate advice about what to eat.

The journey this book will take you on will subtly and irrevocably change your beliefs, your thoughts and your actions relating to food. You will learn specifically and in detail exactly how to visualise for weight-loss success and discover that even scientists agree that visualisation can powerfully increase weight loss and its maintenance. You will also learn how to keep the weight off forever, something very few diet books address correctly. Maintenance diets don't work because they are still diets, but in this programme you will learn ways to naturally speed up your metabolism and techniques that will keep you slim for life, no matter what situation you are in. By the end of this book when you come to A Day in the Life of the New Thin You, you will have achieved so much and will be able to enjoy the success of your new body as well as a newfound normal relationship with food that I and so many of my clients enjoy on a daily basis. You will be rewired to be a normal weight for life, just as you were born to be. You also have an audio download (see Contents page) which will help you keep up all the changes you are going to make. The audio download is designed to reinforce everything this book will teach you so please don't play it until you have finished the book.

Why I Do What I Love and Love What I Do

In my practice of over twenty years I have worked with thousands of clients fighting to control their weight and I have seen great and lasting success. This book offers you the same therapy and the same results from the privacy and comfort of your sofa. For years my clients have asked me to write out my programme because for the first time it is a way to change their body that really makes sense to them and it works. This book contains that effective and easy-to-follow approach. My clients swear by my methods to such an extent that I have never ever had to advertise, they all come along by personal recommendation. When people visibly lose weight everyone wants to know how they did it. It was my success in helping people achieve such dramatic weight loss that led me to become the therapist on *Celebrity Fit Club* in England and then in America. My methods were quoted as the only ones that worked on Channel 4's Supersize vs. Superskinny. I was already known as an expert in the field of weight loss and worked with many high-profile clients from actors to singers to royalty to rock stars, and I still do.

Unlike many experts I can fully empathise with my clients as I spent over twenty years dieting and being obsessed with trying to be thinner but never quite making it. The techniques in this book moved me from someone with a weight problem and a very unhealthy obsession to someone who never gains weight. I eat more food and better food than I ever used to eat but I weigh the least I have ever weighed and have effortlessly stayed at this weight for over ten years without dieting or even thinking about it. I also no longer have the frequent headaches, sinus problems or lethargy that I lived with for years.

I wish I had known then what I know now. I wasted years obsessing about my weight, turning down invitations to dinner parties because the only way I could eat less was not to be around food. I drove my partner crazy because I would not go to office parties or functions in case I ate too much. I was scared of food and had almost no control over my consumption of it and I craved sugar and carbohydrates. I did not know how to be indifferent to food or how to have a healthy and enjoyable relationship with it, but I do now and you will too as you move through this book. I want you to have the same results, the same freedom and the same healthy body and mindset, and I know that you can.

Overeating is so often an emotional issue and dieting can't fix that, but a form of therapy can. This book is that therapy. It's the new and effective way forward in weight control. Following the process in this book will allow you to become and stay slim by making permanent emotional adjustments ensuring you change from the inside as well as changing on the outside. Unlike diets which we abandon when we cannot do them properly or continuously, you are not required to do anything continuously or fanatically. You don't even have to do all of it all the time, as long as you do most of it most of the time you will succeed.

The great thing about making mental changes is that it's free, painless and easy. The adjustments and changes I will ask you to make are often small and simple but the benefits can be huge and life changing. When you are making physical changes there is no doubt the harder you work the better the results. With mental changes the opposite applies, it does not require huge effort or constant and ongoing work, it just requires that you do it and persist in spending a few moments every day reinforcing it in your mind.

You Have a Few Moments Every Day, Don't You?

Many of the mental changes I will introduce can be reinforced when you are lying in the bath, travelling to work, even when you are cleaning your teeth. Since you spend all day thinking and communicating with yourself you are going to continue doing that, only so much more productively. This may be a hypnosis book but it isn't going to send you to sleep, it's going to wake you up.

STEP ONE

Attitude Adjustment to Get Results

What drives us to overeat are feelings: I need it; I must have it: this food will make me feel better. Diets don't stop the feelings. They can only ever briefly suppress them. Since the feelings will always win (one of the rules of the mind is that feelings will *always* overcome logic as they are so much more powerful) it stands to reason we have to change the feelings rather than the diet. This is exactly what you are going to learn to do, by changing the feelings around food and the association certain foods have, those foods will cease to be of interest to you. The opposite of love in this case is not hate, it is indifference – you can become indifferent and uninterested by the very foods that used to run you. You can have a normal relationship with food and a normal body weight for good. You won't have to resist the urge as the urge will no longer be there. You won't have to fight cravings as they'll be gone. It is so empowering to not even want or think about food all the time.

I spent my teens and twenties obsessed with food and preoccupied with trying to be slim but never quite succeeding. Then, when I began to study hypnotherapy while living in Los Angeles, I discovered there is another way, an easier way. Through the ground-breaking discoveries I made over more than twenty years of working with overweight clients, first in gyms as a personal trainer and nutritionist, and later as a therapist on television, the radio and in my own clinic, I devised a better way to show people that they don't have to be overweight and they don't have to be miserable by taking up one diet then another with no end in sight. You will find my methods very different – you will also find that they work.

It is an unfortunate truth that to be overweight you not only have to have a lifestyle that supports it but also a belief system and convictions about your weight which are keeping you the wrong shape and size. These need to be broken. We are all programmed to act and react in certain ways, human behaviour is not random, it's quite predictable. You are simply going to reprogramme your attitude to food so that it is the one you were born with, not the one you have acquired through bad habits and even ignorance in some cases. You were born able to leave food, able to say no to it, able to stop as soon as you were full; regaining that ability is exciting and liberating.

When you were a baby you loved to feed – all babies do – however, babies only eat when they are hungry. If they are tired, unwell or irritable they won't eat. Small children almost never finish food. If you go to any infant school at lunchtime or to a toddlers' tea party you will notice how much food is left uneaten and has to be thrown away. At every small child's party each plate will have on it a half-eaten sandwich, some crisps and a cake that has had only a few bites taken out. Even when you give small children ice cream or chocolate, when they have had enough they will hand the remains back to you.

You did this once. You may not remember, but you did. You came into the world with normal eating habits, free from addictions to sugar, fast food, junk food, sweets and crisps and free from overeating. By being made to finish everything, by being rewarded and consoled with food and by eating the wrong food you have established a negative pattern. You have become conditioned to link food to comfort, love and to feeling good, and you might link guilt to leaving food, but you can undo this quite easily. Your mind remembers how to eat normally and you can reactivate and recreate that through this programme. Since you were born with a healthy and selective attitude to food you don't have to learn anything new, you just need to relearn habits that already exist within you and once you have reactivated them you can keep them for ever.

When you question a belief you start to doubt it and no longer hold it to be true. When working with overweight patients I look at their beliefs. The same beliefs come up over and over again:

- Everyone in my family is overweight.
- I have tried but I just can't lose weight.
- Diets don't work for me.
- I have big bones.
- I have a big skeleton.
- My metabolism doesn't work properly.
- I have been on every diet there is and they never work.

Very rarely are these beliefs true, but if you continue to talk about yourself like this then you are continuing to be a part of the problem instead of being part of the solution. Even if they were true you can change a belief which in turn can change your body, because our beliefs affect the physiological processes in our bodies. Every thought we think creates a physical change in our bodies. Thoughts can affect blood flow, blood pressure, heart rate and your thoughts can affect weight. Channelled properly, motivational thought processes can be more powerful than pharmaceutical drugs. I am going to show you how to change the images, words and beliefs you run in your head on a daily basis and how this in turn is going to change your body and your entire relationship with food.

We Are What We Eat, We Are Also What We Think and Believe

Telling yourself you have been on millions of diets and nothing ever works for you is not true. No one has been on millions of diets.

You have not been on this one before because it is not a diet. And it absolutely will work for you. Permanently.

It's Not Your Fault

All diets are flawed and none can be sustained long term so if you have failed on any diet, join the club. It is not your fault: 98 per cent of all diets fail which means that only 2 per cent, a staggeringly low number of people, can maintain the weight loss by going on a diet. If diets did work, new ones would not constantly crop up to replace the old ones that promised everything and did not deliver or were just too restrictive, rigid and difficult to stick with. Keeping the excess weight off can be as hard and for some people even harder than actually losing the weight. While most dieters lose weight only to gain it all back again, many also gain additional weight too because they resume their old bad habits. They veer from the low-fat diet to the no-fat diet, the low-carb to the no-carb diet. The Cambridge eating plan is superseded by the Australian one, then the French, then the Japanese. Confusing isn't it?

When I became a fitness instructor in 1982 gyms and exercise classes were a new phenomenon. Today there are more gyms, classes and exercise DVDs than ever before, there is more diet advice and yet there are more overweight people than ever before, so something isn't working and that something is dieting. We usually change our eating habits for only as long as it takes to lose weight and frequently give up before we have reached our target. But you can stay at your ideal weight for life if you welcome the changes and feel pleased about your new mindset. By changing from the inside and changing your relationship to food you are much more likely to succeed.

Triggering Change

The first stage in changing our attitude to food is awareness that nothing in life *ever* influences humans more than what they link to pain and pleasure, and then using this information to our benefit. Moving towards pleasure and away from pain is a survival instinct. This means that every single time you experience pleasure your subconscious searches very fast to find the cause of it, your brain then stores the cause of that pleasure and reminds you of it next time it becomes aware you need to feel pleasure. When you experience pain (any pain, physical or emotional) your mind searches even harder for the cause of the pain. It locks onto and remembers that cause (even if you don't) and then does everything it can to stop you moving towards that pain again.

Your brain is programmed to constantly move you towards pleasure and away from pain and it will always do more to avoid pain than it will to find pleasure, because avoiding pain is how we survive. Just think of how nature works with our instincts by making old food lose its appeal when it goes mouldy because it looks so horrible with fluff and mould growing on it that we link pain rather than pleasure to eating it.

If you have ever had food poisoning from eating bad food, in the moment when you are kneeling over the toilet vomiting you will link absolute pain to the food that caused it. You will say things to yourself like, 'Never again. I will never eat shellfish again.' You may even voice this to other people. By this point your brain has clearly linked huge pain to shellfish, and guess what, next time you even so much as smell some it may turn your stomach. Some people can never again look at, smell, touch or be around a food that made them ill.

When I was small if I had a cold my grandmother made me a hot toddy with whisky and encouraged me to drink it down. It was the most disgusting thing. I absolutely loathed the taste of it and to this day I cannot bear the taste of whisky. I would never drink it. If I pour one out for someone else and get any on my fingers I wash it off immediately as I also hate the smell.

When you were eating as a small child you were already setting up pain and pleasure cues with regard to food, and these will still be influencing you as an adult. You will have been rewarded with certain food as a treat and made to eat some food you hated even though you did not consciously choose to link pain and pleasure to them.

I want you to think of a food you simply could not eat and think about why you can't eat it. As you think about why, you will find that in your mind you link pain to eating that food. Since you can already do this you are going to learn to do this with any food you would prefer to be free of. Celebrities, for example, link huge pain to looking fat in photos or on screen and that pain gives them the resolve to eat differently. They link enormous pain to not getting work because they don't look slim. Because they link pain to being seen as fat they also link pleasure to eating selectively and as a result are able to control how, what and when they eat very successfully.

I have been on many shoots and always find the celebrities stay well away from the canteen or the catering trucks. They will request that their food is sent to their trailer or dressing room and avoid being around the huge fry ups and high-calorie food available for the crew. They will request the type of food they want and if it is not on set they will send someone out to get it or bring their own food with them. They avoid temptation because they link pain to looking fat and pleasure to looking slim and this becomes so ingrained in them that they are able to avoid foods that would lead to weight gain. When celebrities are being filmed in their underwear or swimwear or the Oscars are looming and they want to look particularly good they have even more resolve that allows them to restrict how they eat in order to look amazing. The looking amazing is more important to them than eating junk food. You don't have to be so extreme but changing what you link pain and pleasure to will change your whole attitude to food permanently.

It isn't just stars who do this, vegetarians clearly link pain to eating meat and there is no dilemma for them. If they were on a long flight and only meat was available they would eat nothing rather than eat meat. They might improvise with other foods but they could not and would not eat any food they linked pain to. Muslims are taught that pork is dirty so they link pain to it and do not eat it. Orthodox Jews will not eat shellfish for the same reason. The footballers I work with all have a huge enough discipline not to eat stodgy food before a match as it slows them down. They simply link pain to not performing at their best during the game and the pain is linked to any food that could have this effect on them so even if they are around it they won't eat it.

The problems begin when we link pain and pleasure to the same thing. This causes huge problems for our mind; it is confusing for our brain because it can't do what it is designed to do. It can't move us towards pleasure and away from pain when they are linked to the same thing simultaneously. So when you eat sweets and say, 'These are delicious but I shouldn't have them because they make me fat,' you are linking pain and pleasure to the sweets simultaneously, likewise when you eat a cake and say 'This is yummy but it's going straight to my hips'. When you link pain and pleasure to the same item your brain becomes like a spin-dryer going round and round and getting nowhere. This confusion will affect your mindset. If you don't run your brain and take charge of it, your mind will be influenced by advertisers and food manufacturers.

Anorexics and bulimics are affected by exactly this confusion, because what they love they also hate and what they hate they also love. That thing is, of course, food. Anorexics like shopping for food, reading about food, even cooking for others, but they won't eat much at all. I have anorexic clients who go to the supermarket every day and spend hours looking at all the different food and getting pleasure from it, but they always buy the same items: some lettuce, an apple and some tomatoes, because they link pain to eating food that is high in calories. If I ask a bulimic what he or she loves they will say 'I love food, I love junk food, I love eating it, tasting it, smelling it, bingeing on it.' When I ask them what they hate they reply 'I hate having food in my body, I hate being full, I have to make myself sick because I hate it so much.'

I have similar conversations with my clients who are simply overweight. 'What makes you happy?' I ask them. 'Eating, especially eating ice cream and puddings,' they reply. 'So what makes you unhappy?' I continue. 'Well, come to think of it eating ice cream and puddings is making me unhappy. I mean, look at the size of my stomach. How can I be happy with that?' they reply as they prod it in mock horror. 'Well let's get you to stop eating them.' 'Oh no, I don't want to do that. I would miss ice cream so much. I couldn't enjoy going to the cinema without ice cream.' 'So what do you want?' 'I want to be thinner that would make me happy. But I don't want to give up my treats because that would make me unhappy. Have you got any other way?'

Confused? Me too, but I was the same once. When I was at hypnosis school my teacher offered to hypnotise me to stop eating chocolate and I actually refused because I liked it too much. Even when one of my back teeth broke when I bit into some hard chocolate and it cost me £400 to fix it I still didn't link enough pain to chocolate. Here's an example of how the pain–pleasure cues affect your appetite. If you ordered a pizza in a restaurant and were watching the waiter bring it over piping hot and smelling wonderful you would link pleasure to eating it and maybe start to salivate in anticipation. If just as the waiter put it on your table he sneezed all over it you would immediately link revulsion to eating it and would not eat it no matter how hungry you were. You have in an instant reversed what you link pain and pleasure to and this has in turn affected your appetite. The good news is that you can do this permanently with any foods you choose.

> You cannot succeed on any diet loving and hating the same food, wanting it, denying it and then craving it. Think of the foods you love and the foods you hate. You can even write them out in a notebook. You can learn to link pain to the wrong foods, the ones that may have cost you so much in terms of weight gain or lack of confidence, while linking pleasure to enjoying healthy nutritious food. If you link pain and pleasure to the same food – maybe hot dogs, crisps or chocolate – you can make yourself link only pain to them.

Your mind cannot move you towards your goal of being slimmer when you link pain and pleasure to the same thing, i.e. loving a huge slice of cake then hating yourself for eating it. We would hate the idea of eating grubs and insects but if we were starving out in the wilderness somewhere we would eat them, we might even eat them with relish. We might be so thrilled to find some form of food we would fight others for our share of it. In doing so we would change what we link pain and pleasure to. You can do this at any time. I read about an English girl in prison in India. She reported that the daily rice portion contained maggots which she ate as they were her only source of protein. She linked pleasure rather than pain to finding maggots in her food.

On the TV series *I'm a Celebrity Get Me Out of Here* the celebrity contestants had to eat grubs, insects, animal genitalia and fish eyes in order to earn food for their colleagues. They ate this horrible food by linking pleasure to getting food for the other celebrities and because they knew that being seen to do this on television made them heroic to the viewers. They linked pain to failing on television, losing popularity and not getting any food for their campmates. This ability to almost instantly change what they linked pain and pleasure to allowed them to do something that was unthinkable only days earlier.

An example of a similar situation in your life would be if you hate the dentist and avoid going and then find yourself in agony with an infected tooth. If the tooth pain is bad enough you will ring the dentist and beg for an appointment. You will link pleasure to getting an appointment instead of pain. You may even thank the dentist profusely for fitting you in. You may sit in the chair and be so happy to take the injection as it is removing your pain instead of causing it. Again, you will have reversed what you link pain and pleasure to.

Only humans can choose what to link pain and pleasure to. It is a major advantage but it can also become a major disadvantage. A cat cannot choose to link pleasure to having a bubble bath any more than a husky dog could choose to link pleasure to being on a beach in tropical heat. You can choose what to link pain and pleasure to and in doing so you can succeed or fail to have the kind of body and health you want.

If you are very overweight you may need to accept that some foods are addictive and not right for your body, just as other people have to accept allergies or religious restrictions and incorporate them into their diet. It is easier and kinder to yourself because it will make you link pain to the wrong foods which in turn helps you to accept that you don't need them, instead of linking pain to the fact that you can't eat those foods and feeling sorry for yourself because of it. You can link pleasure to your ability to become indifferent to junk food instead of linking pleasure to eating it.

When I was in America filming *Celebrity Fit Club USA* the cook was making us all scrambled eggs for breakfast in accordance with my eating plan. One of the celebrities refused to eat them, and when I asked her why she said 'Eggs give me gas and I never eat them while I am filming as I could not bear to get gas on set, it's too humiliating.' Her ability to link pain instead of pleasure to eating eggs allowed her to refuse them easily without seeing it as a hardship. She saw refusing the eggs as a better choice than eating them.

You have enormous power to choose what to link pain to. Now that you realise just how effective this power can be, use it consciously and to your advantage to link pain to junk food, sugar and fat-laden snacks as well as actually being overweight. At the same time link a lot of pleasure to being slim, having energy, refusing to fill up your body with junk, wearing the kind of clothes you want to wear and feeling sexy.

Everything we want in life, with few exceptions, is because of how we think it will make us feel. Look at the feeling you think you get when you eat junk food and realise you are eating it because you think it will make you feel good. It may make you feel good for a brief period of time when it's in your mouth and stomach, but it will never make you feel good long term. However, you can get the feeling without the food and this book will show you how.

If you keep telling yourself you want chocolate or you need cakes it's because you think the chocolate or cakes will make you feel good or happy or better than you are feeling without them. You can make wanting to be thinner much more important. People who successfully control their weight want to be slimmer more than they want to eat cake. Eating cake or chocolate may make you feel good momentarily whereas becoming your ideal weight will make you feel good for good. Stop telling yourself that eating junk makes you feel better as that simply is not true long term – tell yourself instead that eating selectively and being your ideal weight makes you feel amazing. A good way to do this is to think of the longest time you feel good after eating sugar and then how long you feel good for when you eat properly.

Change Your Language, Change Your Body

- Empty
- Full
- Starved
- Hungry
- Nourished
- Satisfied
- Content
- Fulfilled

These are all emotional words. We can feel emotionally empty, starved of affection, sex starved, hungry for success, nourished by the love of our friends and family and full of love or full of resentment.

When we feel empty we eat to fill that emotional void because the stomach is the seat of all emotions. This means that most feelings originate in the stomach. We experience excitement, fear, panic, nerves, tension and anxiety in our stomachs. We have conditioned ourselves to eat to push the feelings down, to ignore them, to make them go away or because we tell ourselves that the feeling must be hunger when it isn't. If your subconscious mind can misinterpret these words and feelings don't be surprised that you have done the same. Instead of saying to yourself 'I am hungry' whenever you feel anything, ask yourself what you are feeling and deal with the feeling or accept the feeling. There is nothing wrong with feeling sad or stressed, but eating when you feel anything but hunger punishes your body and leads to more stress and sadness. Emotional eating or what I call mood food does not work. Eating when you are stressed does not end the stress, but having a hot drink is beneficial as hot drinks release endorphins in the brain and keep our moods up.

We all know that 'we are what we eat' but most of us don't know that in addition we are what we speak. Our words become our reality and our mind uses the words we speak to identify what we are feeling. Your brain takes every word you say as literal and accurate, so if you say 'I am famished', 'I am starving', 'I am ravenous' or 'I could eat a horse' your brain will believe you are starving and will encourage you to overeat. We have something called an appestat that kicks in when we have eaten enough and tells us we are full. However, if you have already told your brain you are starving or famished then your body will respond by ignoring the appestat and encouraging you to overeat as if you really were in a famine or starving situation. Instead you need to use words which are much less negatively descriptive: 'I could eat now' or 'I am ready to eat now' are much better because they are neutral and don't give your brain the intense message that saying 'I am ravenous' does. Your brain has to accept and act on the words and pictures you give it. The less intense the words and pictures you use are, the less intense will be your relationship with food. So don't use words with a strong negative emotional content or words that create a negative picture in your mind because the more descriptive and negative those words are the more they will increase your negative feelings about your body and how you eat.

Whatever we tell ourselves our mind absorbs and accepts. While your mind is used to filtering and sorting information that is presented to you, it has no capacity to reason with the information or signals you tell yourself, it believes whatever you tell it. Because of this getting into the habit of telling yourself only positive things is extremely effective. You also need to get into the habit of being very aware of the language you use – the words to describe things – most especially to describe yourself, because your mind particularly responds to words and images that are symbolic. The subconscious mind loves descriptive words, words that make an immediate picture.

Here is an example: A client comes to my office and I ask her, 'Hi, how are you?' She responds, 'I'm a train wreck, my bum is the size of a barn, I eat like a pig non-stop and I'm the size of a house. I'm just a hopeless mess and I can't stop eating.'

So how much of that statement is true?

1 She isn't a train wreck.
2 Her bum is not the size of a barn.
3 She has never ever eaten like a pig in her life.
4 She is not the size of a house and never could be.
5 She is not a hopeless mess.
6 She can and does stop eating much of the time.

How much of that statement does her mind believe is true and act upon? Yep, every single word is accepted by her mind as a fact and now her mind is working to make that picture a reality and, because it's such a vivid descriptive image, the mind has an easier job of it. If you say I am huge, I am a big fat pig and my bum is the size of a bus or I could eat a horse, your mind first makes a picture of what that means, and then works to have you feel and act in ways that match the picture you are causing your mind to make. You will overeat if you keep using these descriptions to tell yourself what you are feeling. One of the rules of the mind is that your body *must* act in a way that matches your thinking, it literally has no choice. Since thoughts always come first your mind always influences your body and it can never be the other way round. Language is so involved in this. When people are unhappy they use phrases like 'I feel so low', 'I am so down', 'I am sinking' and their body language is stooped and lowered. When they are happy they use phrases like 'I am so up', 'I am on a high', 'I feel on top of the world', 'I feel brilliant' and their body language is the direct opposite of someone who is down.

Remember, the way you feel is linked to the way you focus, and the way you focus is down to:

1 The pictures you make in your mind.
2 The words you use.

Don't use negative words or pictures. You are not a big fat pig with legs the size of tree trunks and you are not going to refer to yourself like this ever again. There is probably no one in the world you talk to as meanly as you do to yourself. If you spoke to your friends like that they would be long gone. Stop punishing yourself. It is important to remember that criticism withers people and praise builds them up. Praise yourself more and you will find it easier to change.

Make a list of the negative things you say to yourself, similar to the one below, and then change your statements into positive things about yourself and reinforce the changes.

NEGATIVE	POSITIVE
I am absolutely starving	I need to eat something
I could eat a horse	I could eat now
I will always be fat	I am changing my shape and size
I can't leave food/refuse it	I feel powerful when I leave food/refuse it
I am just an out-of-control pig	I know what to do and how to do it now
I am the size of a house	I am becoming leaner every day
I eat as much as ten men	I have a normal selective appetite

Once you have written out your new statements I want you to think about how you are going to use them. For example, if you are about to go out to eat with friends or are choosing a restaurant, even if people around you are saying, 'Let's pick this one, I'm starving', you can still make your own statement by saying 'Let's pick this one as I need to eat something'. In that way you are able to agree with your friends but still make a positive statement that helps you instead of hurting you. If you return home from work each evening and say, 'I am ravenous' as you walk through the door just change that to 'It's time to give my body some healthy food'. Remember, the point of this exercise is to give your body the instructions that you want it to respond to. If you hate leaving food just imagine how great it will be to feel that food has no power over you and how liberated you will feel when you state, 'I refuse to treat my body as a dustbin. Waste food is waste, wherever it goes, it's not going into me,' then leave something on your plate to reinforce that power. If you say, 'I eat non-stop' and really consider that statement you'll see that it isn't true: you don't eat while you are sleeping, showering or using the toilet, so change that statement to 'I eat selectively'. Whatever you have been saying that is negative you can easily flip it over to find the positive and say that instead.

Small Changes, Big Benefits

Fact 1 All human pain is linked to the word loss.
Fact 2 We cannot succeed at weight loss or losing weight.

So what do these two facts add up to? Loss is bad, gain is good. This may sound illogical but it's true: if you want to become leaner, do not use the words 'weight loss' or 'losing weight'.

Loss is one of the most negative words in our vocabulary because the strongest force in the human psyche is to try to get back everything we think we have lost. Clients will often tell me they have lost hope or lost faith or lost their enthusiasm. Some have even lost the will to live. Others describe losing their looks or losing their husband or wife or their freedom or jobs. 'I lost the baby' describes a miscarriage; 'I lost it' means you were not in control. We lost everything in the recession/flood /fire is another one. Companies can go out of business if they lose a client or contract.

Sports people hate to lose as, even in the Olympics, we don't remember who comes second, hence Paula Radcliffe's agony at the Olympics in Greece when she realised she would not win a gold medal. Teenagers describe those they don't like as 'Losers' and even hold up their finger and thumb to make the letter 'L'. It's a form of great insult. When we describe someone as having lost the plot, lost their marbles or lost their mind it's very negative and critical. I once worked with someone who through illness lost his hair, his hearing and his mobility, but when he lost his sight he also lost all his independence and then the will to live. Lossage is an insurance word for loss. Gamblers feel they must regain their loss and will stay in a casino all night losing even more money in an attempt to get back what they have lost.

When people feel they have lost their looks they will try to look the same as they did twenty years ago. Wearing the same styles they wore when they were at their very best makes them feel more in control of the loss. Relationships end when one partner loses their desire or respect for the other. If you keep referring to loss your psyche will try everything to regain what it thinks you have lost. For this reason it is very detrimental to focus on how much weight you have lost or want to lose.

I often ask my clients to list everything good about the word loss and everything negative about the word gain, and it's a very short list. Apart from gaining weight, gain is a good word. We gain status, promotion, wisdom, a family, recognition, a degree, qualifications, skills, a pay rise, gifts, love and riches. It is not easy to find any good losses and negative gains – try it yourself, see if you can think of anything that's good to lose then think of all the things that are so bad to lose. You can write them out yourself and you will be surprised at how few, if any, good losses there are.

Your brain simply cannot accept that all loss is bad but, oh wait, there is one exception: losing weight is good. As far as your brain is concerned *all* loss is bad and gain is very good indeed. Don't fight this fact, work with it and it will work for you.

I get my patients to replace loss with:

- I have let go of 10 pounds.
- I have reduced by half a stone.
- I have shed 10 pounds.
- I have dropped a dress size.
- I have taken off 6 kilos.
- I am dropping weight.
- I am shedding pounds.
- I am becoming leaner/lighter.
- I am becoming a size 12.
- I am becoming a smaller shape/size.
- I am getting back to the right size and weight for me.

Reduced, discarded, shed, let go, dropped, taken off, got off, eliminated and erased have less emotional attachment to them than the word loss. Find another word that works effectively for you and stop talking about losing weight. If you slip up occasionally don't feel bad, just correct the statement with something that works. What image do you associate with the word loss? What picture comes to mind when you think of loss? Usually the association with loss is death, pain, grief – all sad emotions, whereas the pictures you make when you say shed, reduce or discard are not painful at all.

Ownership

Fact 3 'My' is an ownership word. 'My' is also another emotional word.

One of the most forceful rules of the mind is that it is reluctant to give up anything you prefix with 'my'. The clients I work with who have the most severe illnesses and symptoms always talk about *my* headaches, *my* problems, *my* depression, *my* illness, even *my* cancer. The clients who come to see me to shed weight talk about *my* weight, *my* fat, *my* enormous appetite, *my* greed, *my* problems with food, *my* huge stomach, *my* constant hunger.

Never use the word 'my' as a prefix to something you wish to be free of because this makes the mind accept something as belonging to you when it doesn't. The mind finds it much harder to part with or change anything which you continue to refer to as 'my' or 'mine'. Only prefix something with 'my' if you are proud of it and want to keep it. For instance, you can talk about *my* commitment to this programme, *my* determination, *my* enthusiasm, *my* fantastic progress, in the same way you talk about *my* children, *my* home. These are things you are happy and proud to own.

We have all seen small children fighting over a toy or even a chair they were sitting on while screaming 'It's *mine*'. Adults can get just as upset when someone takes *my* seat, *my* place, *my* newspaper. They become very territorial over something they think they own and your mind is doing the same thing all the time, you just may not have been aware of it before, and now you are it can only help you to succeed in reaching your ideal size and weight.

Your fat does not need to be yours. Does it belong to you? Do you call it mine? Do you want to own it forever, or is the real you underneath the fat? If you say, 'It's mine' and I say, 'I can take it off you it isn't going to be yours any more', you aren't going to fight me for it, you're going to say 'Take it all, with pleasure, I don't want it'. When I was a personal trainer I would often say to my clients, 'We can get rid of the flab with this exercise programme' and no one ever replied 'It's *my* flab and I need to keep it'. If a surgeon doing liposuction takes a handful of your flesh he might say, 'I can take some of this fat away'. Your reply might be 'Can't you take all of it away?' because you don't want it. Who would argue with him and say 'No, you can't have it, it's mine'. You are going to pay him a lot of money and endure some pain to have him take it away. You are not going to take the jars of removed fat home to keep because it's yours and it belongs to you. This would be pointless. It is just as pointless and counter-productive to keep calling a habit you don't want and a size you don't want 'mine' while all the time longing to be free of it. If you don't want it, if you don't want to keep it or own it then constantly referring to it as 'mine' is giving your brain very confusing messages.

Therefore you must prefix anything you want to be free of with the word 'the' not the pronoun 'mine' or progressive adjective 'my'. 'The' is a neutral word which is why women hate being called 'the wife' instead of *my* wife as it does not imply pride or connection, it's just ambiguous. As soon as you talk about 'the' weight issue, 'the' excess weight, 'the' big stomach, 'the' pudding, you have no emotion attached to it and it becomes easier to become and stay free of it. Do not talk about 'my fat legs', 'my big bum', 'this fat stomach of mine', 'my greed', 'my weight problem', 'my chocolate addiction'. Stop saying, 'I love *my* chips', 'I need *my* biscuits', 'I have to have *my* puddings'.

If you slip up just correct yourself. You didn't know better before and now that you do you are going to do better all the time.

Using the previous examples write out all the words you are going to use to replace 'loss'. Next, taking note of how you refer to yourself, write out the words you are going to use instead of 'my' and 'mine'.

The opposite of owning it and calling it 'mine' is shown by people who have no responsibility at all for the weight they have become. Many overweight people do not want to take responsibility for their excess weight and instead try miracle pills or diets, jaw wiring or stomach stapling. I was sent one client who, after having her jaw wired, was drinking twelve pints of milk a day. I noticed that she didn't once use the word 'I' but always used 'you', for example, saying, 'You can't leave biscuits', 'You can't not eat chips when they are on your plate'. 'You have to eat when people cook for you'. 'You can't leave the last few sweets'. Eventually I said to her 'Why do you keep saying "you"? I have no problem saying no to biscuits. Let's just talk about you.'

I made her replace 'you' with 'I' and got her to see that by not associating with her behaviour she was not able to recover. As long as she was saying 'you' she wasn't even talking about herself – she was talking about other people just like her. Saying 'you' makes the problem global instead of individual. Making it global is saying everyone does this so I am not at fault. It is making the whole world just like you so you don't have to feel different or responsible. It was no different to saying, 'One can't say "no" to chocolate, or 'One needs puddings to cheer up'.

Another way people disassociate is to refer to themselves as big, for example, 'We are big people so we can't really exercise', or 'I am a big person so I need more food', or 'I come from a big family'. If you are overweight it can be very painful and you certainly don't need more pain but you do need to take responsibility for the words you use to talk to and about yourself. Don't disassociate and talk about what other people do. Let's just make this all about you.

More on Words

The words you use in front of words can dramatically increase and decrease the intensity of your statement. For example, 'I am successful' is more intense when you say 'I am incredibly successful' or 'constantly successful'. 'I love eating like this' is stronger when you say 'I always love eating like this'. 'This eating plan is so easy' is easier still when you say 'this eating plan is so amazingly easy'. Equally, chips become less appealing if you say 'fatty, oily, greasy, lardy chips floating in an oil slick'. Swear words are naturally used to increase the intensity of descriptions so use this to your advantage: 'I look fantastic' is more intense when you say 'I look fan-bloody-tastic', and 'I look so damn amazing' is more powerful than just amazing.

Avoid words like 'try', 'hope', 'wish' or 'dream': 'I am trying to stay on the diet', 'I wish I could be a size 12', 'I dream of being thinner', 'I hope I succeed this time'. These words convince your mind that you have no power or ability to make it happen and that you are depending on some external force to make it work. You are wishing, hoping and dreaming of it working because it is beyond your ability to pull it off.

When you replace the above words with 'I *know*', 'I *can*', 'I *will*', 'I *am*' you immediately move into a 'take charge and succeed' mentality. Put those words into your statements so they read like this: 'I will stay on this diet', 'I absolutely definitely will be a size 12', 'I can be thinner', 'I know I will succeed', and 'I am making it work for me'.

One Last Word – Enough!

I am 'enough' is the most powerful word of all and my absolute favourite. I'll show you just how important this word is, and then how to go about using it for its maximum impact.

I had been working with people with eating issues for several years and was very struck by the fact that they could never seem to get enough to eat and never felt they were enough in themselves as people either. It wasn't hard to make a connection and the connection became clearer with every overweight person I saw for therapy.

Overeating generally stems from an inner feeling of lacking something and emptiness. One of my clients described it to me as a feeling of being hollow inside. Therefore we need more food and more material things to compensate for the lack we feel and to fill the void within us. Instead of filling that void with food and purchases you need to understand that the void exists only in your mind and you have the power to close it forever. The unconscious need to be physically bigger, to be substantial to stand out and be noticed often stems from feeling insignificant in childhood. Many of my clients have become physically bigger than they ever wanted to be because when they were little they felt insignificant or small.

**When you know and believe you are enough you don't
need more.**
   **When you feel and believe you are not enough you will
always want more.**

A few years ago I worked with Richard, a very successful actor who kept gaining weight and losing out on acting roles because of it. During hypnosis it emerged that Richard's father would eat a full cooked dinner every night while his son had beans on toast at the same table. His father always had nicer food than him and much more of it. Richard was never offered any of his father's food. The family had little spare money and, as the breadwinner and a manual labourer, Richard's father felt he was entitled to eat hearty meals while his son was not. This scenario was played out over and over. At Sunday lunch his father had the biggest helping and any second helpings were always given to the father. I asked him 'Did your father ever give you any leftovers?' He replied 'There rarely were any but if there were he would sooner give them to the dog than me.' The message Richard picked up by being given inferior food or smaller amounts was that he was not good enough and that even the dog was more worthy than him.

In my experience when people feel they are not enough they go into a mental state of 'lack' and just cannot get enough. Often this manifests itself by them never feeling they have had enough to eat, always wanting more food, worrying that the food will run out, eating like there is no tomorrow and doing it all again a few hours later.

When I said to Richard, 'You just don't ever feel you are enough, do you?' huge tears welled up in his eyes and he cried. He then said, 'I never thought of it like that before but it's true.' I made Richard repeat to himself out loud every waking hour 'I am enough'. He stuck some notes on his mirror, car dashboard, fridge and screensaver with the same message and reminded himself of this truth every day until it stuck.

In Richard's case the drive to be more and the need to eat more stemmed from his core feeling of never being enough. This had made him become a very successful actor because he wanted and needed everyone to see him as something and someone, but he never believed it of himself and was very unhappy and overweight because of it.

I cannot emphasise enough how important it is to tell yourself you are enough. It is so simple but the results can be life changing. You must say 'I am enough' constantly. Say it out loud. Say it with feeling. Say it like you mean it and say it over and over again and do so for weeks until it sinks in and replaces the feeling that you are not enough, which may be driving you to overeat. This will make you feel enough, whereas overeating will not. Begin and end every day with the words:

'*I am enough*', and '*I am always enough*', '*I am more than enough*', '*I have enough*'.

Write it on your screensaver, your mirror, stick a note on your wallet and your fridge, write it on your hand if it helps and repeat it to yourself over and over and really get it because *it's true*!

Saying 'I am enough' before eating is particularly helpful as it can really curb your appetite and remove the desire to overeat. Say it at the end of every meal as well to confirm that you don't need more. You can say it in your head when you are with company but say it out loud whenever you can. If you find yourself munching away on bags of nuts or any portable food just put them down and remind yourself 'I am enough, I don't need these'.

Many people when they first fall in love totally lose their appetite. During the first flush of love when they are constantly told by their partner 'I love you, you're amazing, you're the best', they do feel enough, they believe it will be like this forever and their hunger diminishes because they are so nourished emotionally. When I met the love of my life I knew it was the real thing because we went away together for the weekend and both of us had no desire to eat at all. I knew women did that but I was amazed and secretly thrilled that he did the same.

At this point you might be wondering how such a method can really work, especially if when you repeat 'I am enough' to yourself you find your mind coming up with all kinds of objections such as 'I am not really enough, I have cellulite and I can't wear stylish clothes'. At this stage many people give up not realising that it is *you* who is coming up with the objections and *you* who has the power to stop them. To fix that for good, counter the objections like this: 'Yes I have cellulite, and I am still enough,' and 'I will wear stylish clothes even sooner as I accept I am enough'.

Then 'I am not enough or I wouldn't be alone' becomes 'I am enough and I don't have to be alone'. And 'How come I don't have a boyfriend if I am enough?' becomes 'My fears kept men away, but as I accept I am enough so will any man I get involved with. The more I like me the more they will like me.' And 'I am always hungry' becomes 'I feel full, nourished and satisfied by so many things other than food.'

It's natural initially to come up with objections to the 'enough' affirmations – what you need to do is look at the objections and shoot them down with something better. If you are determined and keep on with the affirmations, eventually you will run out of objections and your mind will conclude, 'You say this so often and with such conviction it must be true' and with that your mind is agreeing with you and you are finally making real progress. Now you are becoming a physical expression of what you believe

I am enough instead of becoming a physical expression of the opposite: I am not enough.

A few months after my session with Richard I was walking towards my gym and saw a man ahead of me on the street. As I got nearer he seemed to recognise me and started to undo his trousers and lift up his shirt. I wondered what on earth was going on and as I got closer I realised it was Richard. He said, 'Look, my stomach is flat now, look how much weight I have lost, look at that', and he patted his very flat stomach with absolute pride while walking right up to me so I could admire it too. He told me he had shed three stone. He was beaming. I told him I was thrilled for him but it might not be the best thing to start undoing his flies in the street as a woman approached him. We both laughed and his happiness was infectious.

Choose to Be Thinner

This probably sounds ridiculous to you, but you can choose to be thin by choosing to think and behave differently around food, by choosing to believe different things about food and about your relationship with it.

Choosing to do the right thing is very good for humans as it makes us move towards our goals. Humans are all built as goal-seeking creatures. With goals we have purpose and direction, without them we drift and flounder. Having a goal, taking steps towards its accomplishment and seeing it through to its end makes us feel good about ourselves. Achievement makes us feel satisfied, more self confident and self motivated, more like winners. Having some self control is very liberating. In our Western lives, eating at random anything and everything is not always a freedom; it can imprison us. The unfair reality about being overweight is that overweight people show the world their weakness. They are no weaker than someone who has an addiction to shopping, pain killers, cigarettes, drugs, porn or internet sex, but other addictions can be hidden, disguised or laughed off. Confessing to work colleagues 'I was so fed up I went crazy and overspent on my credit card or drank too much' will illicit murmurs of sympathy, understanding or even humour. However, saying 'I was so down I ate four cakes, two sandwiches and then loads of chocolate until I could hardly move', or saying, 'I ate until I felt sick', can produce revulsion in others.

Because overweight people wear their weakness and we all see it, because they cannot hide it or disguise it, we judge them as weak, as gluttons, as having no control. It is very unfair and cruel but we are an outwardly visual (a lookist) society. We forgive celebrities for being drunk, we even seem to forgive them for using drugs, but we don't seem to forgive them for being fat, and they know it. Paris Hilton's career was enhanced when a film of her having sex was released but it would no doubt end if she became very overweight. Celebrity magazines make a point of highlighting celebrities who have gained weight and mocking them. The message they send is that being overweight is something to be ashamed of but other failings are more acceptable. We are scared of weak people because we are all scared of our own weaknesses and scared of being identified as being like them, so it follows that most people who are critical of fat people are scared of becoming that way themselves.

Fortunately, by making the right choices and using your power of choice you can succeed fully in beating being overweight, reaching your ideal weight and maintaining it. The minute you say 'I can't eat that', 'I mustn't have it', 'I am not allowed it', or 'I should not eat it' you are likely to want it even more as you are trying to deny a desire. Replacing the 'I can't' with 'I am choosing not to eat that' makes an assertion to your mind that you have a choice and are making the right choice willingly. This means you are not using willpower to fight desire, which is usually unsuccessful, but you are using a stronger desire and you will succeed.

In the same way you can say 'I am choosing to eat fruit', or 'I am choosing to leave food on my plate' instead of saying 'I can't eat what I want so I'll have to have this other boring stuff instead' and 'I can't waste food'. Replacing the words 'I can' or 'I can't' with 'I choose to' or 'choose not to', will give you control, power and lasting success. In doing this your brain moves immediately to what you are choosing to do and believes you want to do this so you feel empowered and in control. Studies of very successful people find that they don't say 'I can' or 'I can't'. Successful people say 'I choose to' or 'I choose not' to instead. You can choose to say 'no' to filling up your body with junk food, pesticides and preservatives and 'yes' to slimness.

At the same time you are moving away from denial and resistance. When you constantly refer to what you can't or must not or should not do you literally increase the desire you are trying to deny. Have you ever noticed that when you are on an aeroplane and they lock the toilets an hour before landing that the minute you know you can't go you want to go and the more you try to deny it the harder it is?

When I worked on *Celebrity Fit Club USA* some of the celebrities were very pampered and unused to doing anything that was hard or painful. As they went on the treadmill or running machine for the first time they would, within minutes, start to say 'I hate this' or 'it hurts, it's painful' or 'I don't like it, when can I stop?' The minute we begin to speak in this way our brain begins to look for a way to stop the activity. But saying, 'I am choosing to do this because I am choosing to be thinner so I might as well choose to enjoy it', helps to stop any resistance. You don't even need to lie. When I was a personal trainer in LA and teaching boot camp classes I would always get my class to say, 'My body loves this, my body is benefiting from it, my body likes it', and that was true – they may not have liked the fiftieth sit up but their bodies really did. You would not consider running a marathon while telling yourself after the first mile, 'I hate this and I want to go home'. You would tell yourself, 'I can do it, I will do it; I am doing it' because that would keep you going. When squaddies or marines are training they don't bitch and moan about the exercises, they sing and inspire each other to keep going. By singing and joking through endurance training they are sending a very clear signal to their brain that says 'I have a choice here, I am choosing to do this and choosing to feel good about doing it'.

If you go to the gym and tell yourself you hate it, if you eat salads while telling yourself you hate them you will quickly go back to your old destructive behaviour. Tell yourself you love the gym, tell yourself that your body loves exercise (what a concept, actually telling yourself and your body the truth!). By repeating this over and over you will spend more time working out. Tell yourself your body loves fruit and even if it is not true it will become true. If you eat a big salad while saying, 'Yuk this is tasteless rabbit food' you will have no incentive to eat healthy food. Find healthy food that you like and tell yourself, 'My body loves this, I can feel it doing me good'. Even if this isn't an absolute fact it will become one very quickly. If your weakness is chocolate or fry ups tell yourself, 'I am choosing not to fill up my body with fat. I am choosing not to clog up my arteries with grease.'

If a certain food made you ill or brought you out in a rash or made you itch horribly you could look at the food and no matter how good it looked or smelled you would choose not to eat it because it would not be worth feeling ill or coming out in a rash. It would not be hard because your mind would be quite clear about why you made your choice. You wouldn't feel too deprived by its absence. You will be able to get your mind to feel like this about any food by the end of this book as long as you do the exercises.

While doing research for this book I came across some studies from Great Ormond Street Hospital about how epileptic children cannot metabolise flour. One of my clients has a daughter with epilepsy and she decided to try her on a flourless diet. The results were very impressive but her daughter Karen hated the exclusion diet. I was talking to the little girl and she said, 'I can't eat cakes and muffins like my friends,' and I replied, 'Well Karen you can if you want to. You can eat all those things but you don't want to have fits and to have to wear a crash helmet in school so you have to choose what's more important to you. What do you want more, to eat the cakes or to not wear the crash helmet and not have fits?' I know that sounds like a harsh conversation to have with an eight-year-old but it made her feel better, it made her feel like she was choosing to get better rather than having her parents force a diet onto her without her agreement.

People who don't smoke don't say, when offered a cigarette, 'I can't' or 'I shouldn't' or 'I mustn't', they say 'I don't smoke' and it is so easy to refuse something you have chosen not to indulge in. If you don't take drugs or drink spirits, if someone offers them to you, you say no easily because you don't want them, there is nothing for you to deny or resist and in saying no to them you are simply stating a fact.

It's really important for you to know that you can eat whatever you want to but are choosing not to. Very young children and people who are naturally thin do not think about food all day, they only think about food when they are ready to eat. They have no problem refusing food or leaving some food because they have a mindset that says 'I can have this whenever I want it and it will always be available for me' so they often don't want it. It's only when you get into the mindset of 'this is not allowed, I can't have it, it's forbidden' that you want it so much more. In the womb everything we want is available to us and we are born with a belief that food will always be there – with no need to drive or overeat.

Sometimes simple changes have the most powerful results. Actively choosing reminds your mind that you do have a choice. You can choose to be in control rather than being controlled by food. By choosing how to communicate with yourself, how to control your thoughts and how to say and think the right things about how you eat and how you exercise, you really can also choose to be thin. Once you know that you can choose to be thinner you can start to understand that every time you eat pizza and chips followed by cake you are choosing to remain overweight. If you choose to eat fruit instead of a dessert you are choosing to become slimmer. As you accept this fact you also accept that you have not failed at dieting and you are not destined to be overweight or ruled by food. You have been making the wrong choices and choosing to believe you just can't help it, but from now on you can choose not to believe that any more. You have not failed at diets, diets have failed you.

How to Get What You Want

So how much do you want to be slim and what are you willing to do to look and feel the way you want to look and feel? What are you willing to pay to be a normal size? Whatever your answer is you are probably already paying much more by being overweight. If you want to get thin and stay thin for life you have to make a choice: you can either have a diet that is slightly restrictive and a life that isn't, or you can have an unrestricted diet and eat whatever you want whenever you want and pay the price by living a life that is restricted because of your weight. Having experienced both the former and the latter, I promise you the former is better in every way. I have worked with thousands of clients who learned my methods and I frequently get letters thanking me for showing them the way. I have never met anyone in my career of twenty plus years who said, 'I was happier before and I preferred my old eating habits'.

If eating indiscriminately and immoderately made you happy you would be happy by now and you're not. No one who is overweight is truly happy because the price they pay is so horribly high. Being overweight doesn't mean you aren't loveable or wonderful or a great person, but it does mean you are suffering when you don't need to.

I am always amazed when people tell me that they refuse to

restrict their eating while their life is in fact restricted by being overweight. Cutting out certain foods may seem restrictive, but if your weight limits your ability to be happy with what you look like and your self esteem, to be active with friends or family, to buy clothes that you admire on the hanger or in magazines or even affects your sex life, that is truly restrictive. Clients often tell me that they refuse to get involved in the tyranny of restricting what they eat but they are already involved in the tyranny of being overweight. They tell me they refuse to suffer by denying themselves certain foods while explaining how much they are suffering physically and emotionally from being overweight because so many options and activities aren't open to them. They cannot get involved in many activities because they get breathless, they can't play with their children because they are too out of shape. They won't go to the beach, the swimming pool or even a communal changing room because they feel inhibited by their body shape. They can't wear the clothes they want to wear.

You may see eating differently and changing your lifestyle as being enslaved to some dull monotonous diet, but what I'm suggesting is not a diet in the traditional sense at all, and if you aren't leading a full life and don't feel good about yourself and your body then you are already leading a very restricted life and missing out on so much. Restrict your eating instead of your living is a motto I live by, and I should know as I had an eating disorder for years and now I willingly restrict what I eat and I love getting the most out of my life as a result. I have been asked many times if I think my way of eating is restrictive and the honest answer is, yes it is, but only very slightly, whereas being overweight is restrictive all the time. It is much more restrictive to hate your body and to be depressed about how you look and to live life to only half its potential. I feel good almost all the time now, whereas when I was eating without any restriction I felt horrible almost all the time, including when I was eating like there was no tomorrow. I didn't just feel bad about myself and my lack of control, I felt horrible physically, with constant headaches, lethargy, mood swings and stomach aches. And as for the guilt, yes there was an abundance of that too, and no amount of chocolate or ice cream could cure it. If you choose to willingly and happily restrict how you eat, this one action will free you from being restricted in other areas of your life forever, you will never look back with any regrets

What's Restrictive Anyway?

You are probably sick of the 'R' word already, but here's the thing – you already happily live with a wide range of restrictions without a second thought. If you are married you have to accept certain restrictions – you can't behave like a single person, you can't do just whatever you want, come in whenever you want, buy whatever you want and flirt with whoever takes your fancy as you made a choice when you got married to forgo those things. If you have a job you can't go to work whenever it suits you and stay in bed when it doesn't, you can't even wear what you like. Again, in order to keep that job you have to restrain some urges and impulses. We all know that having children means sacrificing late nights, long lie-ins and pristine houses and we make that choice willingly when we want a baby. When you finally get to buy your own home, owning it means you may no longer have surplus cash to spend, but you are willing to accept restrictions in your lifestyle and spending in order to be a home owner and get on the property ladder. Even having pets has almost as many restrictions as benefits especially when it comes to travelling or cleaning up their mess or taking the dog out for a walk when it's pouring and you have the flu, but we accept that it's part of the deal. Nothing comes with only benefits not even that gorgeous puppy or cute kitten.

In terms of restrictions on food, we don't eat garlic or onions if we are about to go on a hot date or go to an interview. We may choose to avoid foods that give us gas like beans, pulses and dried fruits if we are in certain situations such as an important meeting.

These are choices that people willingly make and it is not hard at all with some effort and persistance to transfer these thoughts and feelings to your everyday diet.

With our jobs, pets and relationships we accept the restrictions and enjoy the benefits, and by using this programme to apply the same principles to how you eat you will succeed in reaching and maintaining your ideal weight. Most of us don't abandon our job, spouse or children because they aren't perfect, yet people abandon diet after diet because they can't do it perfectly, we lose motivation as soon as it goes wrong and give up. This is the major flaw with diets – we can never adhere to them completely so we give up and feel like a failure. This programme will work for you because you don't have to do it perfectly in order to get visible and lasting results, you just have to do it.

When I first began to work with overweight clients I was amazed that they would do almost anything to lose weight except change how they ate. They would pay for liposuction, diet pills, crazy quick-fix diets, expensive gym membership that they never used, slimming treatments that were a con and drugs that hadn't been approved and yet they would not embrace a lifestyle where chocolate was an occasional item instead of a regular one. They would even say, 'I would do anything to lose weight', but that turned out not to be the case.

I had many discussions with clients who would begin the consultation by saying, 'It's so unfair that I can't just eat whatever I want'. They had never considered that half the people in the world can't eat whatever they want and even in the developed world many people can't eat whatever they want either due to medical conditions, religious beliefs or financial restrictions. I can't eat whatever I want *and* have the body and good health I want and I accepted that long ago, and once I had accepted it life got better and easier and I became much happier too. Smokers and drinkers can choose to smoke and drink whatever they want, but they know they will ultimately pay a price. So I answered my clients by saying, 'You can eat whatever you want, if you are prepared to pay the price.' I got one client to list what he would have to pay and what he was prepared to pay, and when he saw how high the stakes were he changed his mindset. It was very important that he did it, rather than me forcing it on to him, because we resist being made to do things by others, but are more open to changing when it's our own idea.

When I asked one of my clients to write out what she was paying to eat indiscriminately the list was scarily long. She began with her fertility as being overweight by even a small amount can be linked to polycystic ovary syndrome, and excess fat acts as a kind of sponge absorbing the female hormones vital to conception. She included in her list high blood pressure, heartburn and feeling inhibited when she was naked so she never had the kind of unabandoned sex that both she and her husband would have liked. She ended the list with a higher risk of developing some cancers and her depression about never wearing the clothes she wanted to wear and always feeling that she was missing out.

At the end of this chapter I want you to write out your own list. I don't want to scare you, I'm not a terrorist therapist, but to show you how high the stakes are, what you are paying, what it's costing you, and why it's time to do something different so you can be different. No one reaches the end of their lives and wishes they had eaten more biscuits and cakes. Generally people wish they had done more, seen more and led fuller, richer lives. Overeating is not going to move you towards this, it is going to move you further away from it.

So many of my clients tell me that going to the cinema or theatre isn't as enjoyable as it could be as the seats are too small and uncomfortable and they cannot face the humiliation of having to squeeze past the row of people to reach their seats, knowing they could not go through that again if they needed the toilet halfway through the performance. This is restriction; cutting out the wrong food is a piece of cake by comparison.

Another of my clients who was overweight complained that his wife of only one year was not interested in him sexually. She in turn told me that she still loved her husband but because of his junk food diet he had constant indigestion and loud gas that woke her up at night. She had made a decision to have separate bedrooms because although she loved him he had lost all sex appeal for her. That is a huge price to pay. I had another client who was so depressed about being overweight that it affected his sex drive and made him feel insecure about his body. He didn't want to have sex with his wife who suffered with him because she felt unloved and rejected by him.

For years I tried using food to make me feel better but it never worked and a lot of the time I was absolutely miserable. I love to eat but I have taught myself to love eating the foods my body can digest, that keep me slim and happy. It is so easy now and such a way of life that I wish I had done it years ago. I wasted so much of my twenties dieting then breaking the diet and I didn't have a normal attitude to food because I was preoccupied with losing weight. It's ironic that now I do have a normal attitude to food I actually eat more than I ever ate back then, and I am the weight I always wanted to be.

It is unfair that overweight people cannot enjoy certain every-day foods like snack foods, wheat products like breakfast cereals, and cheese because, as you will see as you read on, they are quite definitely linked to excess weight. It is also unfair that diabetics, people at risk of heart disease, people with high cholesterol and people with nut or fish allergies can't eat at random either. They have to make a choice and eat selectively. But when you know the facts it's easy to appreciate that eating less of the unsuitable types of food for life is much less restrictive and much less of a hardship than being overweight for life. People who have shed weight all readily agree that life is easier when you maintain your ideal weight. All the celebrities and everyday people I have worked with conclude, without exception, that changing how they eat perma-nently, by restricting some foods in their diet in order to be free from the limitations of excess weight is most definitely worth it.

I am not recommending either the usual type of diet where

you have to be so controlling over what you eat, or suffer hunger pangs or a massive deprivation of food, which makes people absolutely miserable. I am recommending eliminating or restricting some indigestible, unhealthy foods that seem to cause weight gain and disrupt weight reduction in many people. There are still so many wonderful, delicious foods you can enjoy. You don't have to give up any food forever, just restrict their intake. I still enjoy rice pudding and rhubarb crumble with custard, but I save them for holidays and high days. I don't need them very often and I don't miss them at all.

Athletes make food choices all the time. Bodybuilders eat more protein and much less carbohydrates so their muscles show more easily. Many bodybuilders restrict their diet six days a week by only eating low-carbohydrate and low-fat foods and then eat anything they like on the seventh day. Actresses and dancers all make food choices and choose to restrict what and how they eat in order to look and feel a certain way. The many celebrities I work with would all admit to willingly restricting their diet in order to reach their dreams and goals and look a certain way. A lot of singers have to forgo all dairy products as the mucus reaction they get from milk affects their voice. The casein in milk triggers histamine production. This in turn triggers mucus production. The mucus collects in the throat, chest and sinuses and blocks the production of sound for singers who use the diaphragm to sing.

Many people choose to restrict how they eat in order to look and feel a certain way. Making a decision and coming to accept that there are certain foods you cannot eat, or cannot eat very often, will help you adapt to a lifestyle of choice that will work for you permanently. Eventually these foods won't even look or seem like food to you. You will find you can be around them without being tempted at all. You will be able to look at, say, doughnuts or cheese and feel indifferent to them.

Behavioural experts have stated that humans do so much better when they are able to accept something rather than fighting it. Accepting it means you will work with it instead of resisting it. By the end of this programme you will be able to accept and embrace a new attitude towards what and how you eat and you will be able to reach and keep your ideal weight for life.

How Much Does It Cost You to Eat Cheap Food?

So far we have been looking at what being overweight is costing you in terms of lifestyle and health but it can also cost a lot of money to be overweight. Generally, people overeat cheap foods like chips, bread, snacks and chocolate and convince themselves that they can't afford to eat any other way. This is not true. We can still eat inexpensive food and shed weight. Fast food isn't cheap in the long run and although we can buy a bag of chips or a bar of chocolate for less than the cost of fresh fruit and vegetables, in the long run we pay dearly for buying cheap food. I have clients who tell me they can't afford to eat anything but fast food yet taking some hard-boiled eggs or tuna with some pitta bread and fruit to work costs less than eating in fast food restaurants. One client I talked to said that after a lifetime spent eating fast food because she told herself she could not afford the alternative, she then ended up paying over £5,000 for liposuction.

The irony is that junk food and processed food are very cheap but they cost you a lot in hidden costs. Being overweight will cost you a lot of money in increased life insurance. Overweight people can pay twice, even three times as much for life insurance and your health insurance premiums will triple – that's assuming you can get insurance. Many overweight people can't get any health insurance at all

Even holding onto a stone of excess body fat unleashes free radicals and triggers inflammation which accelerates ageing and poor long-term health. Hormones released in fatty deposits raise the risk of getting cancer especially for those of us who store fat around the waist. In apple-shaped people (those who store fat around the waist), the fat can press up against vital organs and blood vessels increasing blood pressure and the risk of strokes. Because being overweight brings with it a risk of horrifying related illnesses insurers expect the overweight to have poor health and will load their premiums accordingly. They also expect overweight people to die earlier.

Eating cheaply costs you a lot in the long term. It costs you hugely in terms of your quality of life, your happiness and your relationships. An obsessive relationship with food and an addiction to food will almost certainly disrupt other relationships, most importantly those with your children and partner. It will cost you in terms of your self esteem, your love life, your sex life, your assertiveness, maybe even your career aspirations. If you look long, hard and honestly at what being overweight is costing you, you will understand that eating cheaply is a false economy and is costing you everything.

I want you to spend at least five minutes really doing this and giving it 100 per cent. Ask yourself what it is costing you to eat the way you are currently eating? What will it go on costing you? What price are you paying when you overeat? Are you prepared to pay that price? What are you missing out on?

I want you to really think about your answers and *write them down*. Make a list of what it is costing you, writing down all the illnesses you may have to face and writing out all the emotional and financial costs. Write out what you feel you are missing out on.

Keep going until you have exhausted your answers and then read through your list again and decide if you are prepared to pay that price or if you are ready for a new mindset, one that will work for you rather than against you. If you continue to overeat you are taking a gamble, and sadly the dice are loaded against you.

Once you've finished your list, I want you to focus on the next exercise. Don't just read it and move on. You must *do* it. This is not just a book for you to read, it's a book for you to use. If just reading a book worked you could read a diet book and get results. The results you will get from this programme will come about as a result of you processing the information and doing the exercises. Fully participating in them forms part of that process. So for real results, read through the next paragraph, memorise it and then go back and do it and do it fully, give it 100 per cent and that's what you will get back.

Close your eyes and imagine you can go inside your body and look at all the damage you have done to it by eating badly. Imagine you can see the damage done to your arteries, heart, liver and joints by being constantly stressed from excess food. Look at all the undigested junk food clogging up your stomach and intestines. As well as looking at the physical damage think of the emotional damage you are inflicting on yourself and how eating badly affects your moods and consequently your relationships.

Ask your body how it feels to be treated like this, to be punished like this on a regular basis. Your poor body is working hard every day to keep you alive, well and functioning. How are you repaying it? How does it feel from your body's point of view to be treated with absolute disregard and to suffer unnecessarily on a daily basis? Does your body want to have deal with this every day when you have so much power to change it?

Ask your body to tell you how it really feels about the way you eat and the price it is paying so that you get the message loud and clear. The answers will come to you very clearly if you stay with it and give yourself a little time.

Your body would never ask you to eat like this. The cravings don't start in your body because it hates being overfed with indigestible, processed food. Your body would prefer not to have to work so hard, so unnecessarily. The cravings come only from your mind, and the good news is that since it's *your* mind you can change these cravings for good and you are already doing so as you work your way through this book. Your body is like a small baby depending on you to put the right food in it and paying the price when you don't, so make a commitment to your body that you will look after it and respect it from now on.

Nothing you can ever eat, will ever eat or have ever eaten can give you that satisfying feeling of being a normal weight, liking your body and looking good in your clothes. Being able to put on a pair of jeans or trousers or a little black dress, wearing beachwear without cringing, not having to wear jackets in the stifling heat to cover up, buying clothes off the peg from any shop and knowing they will fit and you will look good in them – is a wonderful feeling. Even more so if you have not experienced it before. It's a feeling you cannot and will not ever find in food.

Enjoying good food is delicious and eating with friends is a wonderful thing, but you cannot find lasting comfort, companionship and joy in food. If you could, believe me, you would have done so by now. Instead, it is more likely that you have become excluded from so much, including activities, relationships, careers and mostly from living a full, long and active life due to poor body image and poor health.

One of my clients had never worn boots in her life because her legs were too large so I asked her to imagine becoming slimmer and then buying some boots, trying on different styles and fashions and looking good in them. I next asked her to imagine being in a restaurant or food shop and trying to find a food that could give her the same feelings she got from imagining wearing the boots. She looked for a long time before she told me there was no food that could match it. Another client had never been able to buy a pair of jeans and when she finally could fit into jeans she was so ecstatic she bought three different pairs. She had never found that ecstatic feeling in any food; she had never even come close to it.

I want you to do one more exercise for me. These exercises are designed to safely change the neural pathways in your brain, which will change your attitude to food. Please take the time to do them rather than just reading them as the effects are very powerful and a key part of this programme. Again, read through and memorise the next exercise then do it.

Close your eyes and imagine you are now at your ideal weight. You look and feel wonderful. You are going into a beautiful store, walking to the clothing department and picking something you have always wanted to wear. It's your ideal size, you try it on it's a perfect fit. You look and feel sensational. You feel so good as you catch sight of yourself in the mirror so you buy it and wear it out of the store. On the way out you go to the food hall. I want you to imagine walking up and down the aisles stopping to look at all the bread and cakes moving on to the chocolate then the sandwiches and snacks then the hot food section, take your time and linger over the food that you think is your favourite. I want you to see what you can find food wise that could give you the same feeling as being your perfect size in your perfect outfit.

After a while you will notice there is <u>nothing</u>, no food at all, that can <u>ever</u> give you that feeling. Even if you could find some food that would make you feel as good as the feeling of being your ideal size it would not last, you would have to keep eating it all the time. We've already been there, done that, this is the new you.

Most of my clients realise this very quickly, while some spend ages mentally considering all the different

---

types of food until they too realise that there is *nothing* you can eat, will eat or have ever eaten that can make you feel as good as you will feel when you like your body. It also helps to work out how long you feel good for after eating say chocolate or pizza and how long you feel good for when you love the way you look. Most of my clients tell me that when they eat sweets or stodge they might feel good for a few minutes, perhaps for as long as they can taste the food in their mouth and feel it going into their stomach and then the feeling is gone. It never lasts that long and it isn't worth it long term. When you like the way you look the feeling will last all day.

Eating gives us instant gratification but it is so in the moment it doesn't last. Eating junk food is ultimately very unsatisfying because it's full of chemicals and additives which are addictive and leave us wanting more. Most people who overeat are very unhappy about it. Sure they are happy while they are tasting the food in their mouths and feeling it go into their stomachs but that feeling doesn't last long. The despair, the self loathing, the feeling of being trapped and the embarrassment last so much longer. Interestingly, one of the definitions of madness is doing the same thing over and over again while expecting a different result. You are ready to do and think differently and you will get a different result, permanently.

So end the exercise by working out how long you feel good for after you have eaten badly and how long you will feel good for when you look the way you want to look. Now go ahead and really do the exercise so you can discover this for yourself. Imagine yourself in detail at your ideal weight, how you'd look and feel and how people would see you.

You Will Always Have Another Day to Eat Cake

You will always have another day to eat cakes, chocolate and biscuits but you only have a certain amount of time to wear the things you want to wear and do the things you want to do. When you are ninety you can eat as many chocolates and crisps as you want to but it will be too late to wear tight jeans, fitted tops, shorts and anything else you are longing to fit into. It will also be too late to do many of the activities you might be putting off as you wait to get thinner – things like running, dancing, cycling and skiing. Putting some restrictions on yourself is not going to take anything away from you; it's actually going to give you so much more back. You won't feel deprived because you will be so focused on all the benefits coming your way.

I am not virtuous. I still eat chocolate sometimes, I enjoy desserts occasionally, I like chips with salt and vinegar, and I enjoy warm bread on the odd occasion but I don't see them as everyday foods. I used to find it really hard to resist chocolate and desserts, but what worked for me was reminding myself that I have all my life to eat them. I was in a restaurant several years ago when I was handed the dessert menu. It listed rhubarb crumble – my favourite. I was thinking along the lines of, 'I have to order this, it's my favourite', when I stopped and told myself, 'I have all my life to eat rhubarb crumble. I can buy it in a supermarket any time I choose and when I am eighty I can eat it every day. I don't need to eat it today just because it's on the menu.' That really worked for me and was a sign that I was succeeding in taking control of how I ate.

It is important to remind yourself that you will always have another day to eat. Many of my clients tell me that when they are confronted with cakes or sweets they eat them as if they will never come across them again. They are at a party with birthday cake, or a friend comes over with chocolate, or their partner brings home a pizza, and they say things to themselves like, 'I have to eat this because it's here, it's free, it's my favourite, etc.'

What works is to tell yourself something different like, 'I have all my life to eat a piece of pizza/cake/chocolate. This is not the only time I am going to be offered it. It's not free, it will cost me a lot to eat it'. That thinking will also allow you to eat a little of something and then put it away. Knowing you can eat it whenever you choose to will stop you finishing everything in front of you just because it's there.

Pizza, cake, biscuits and chocolate are so cheap you will never be denied them and eating them as if you might be is crazy. It isn't going to get you to your ideal weight either. You don't need to eat biscuits just because they are given away free, you have the rest of your life to eat them. For years after I gave up eating sweets I would still take some if they were offered and put them in my bag then put them in a tin when I got home. In doing this I didn't ever feel that I couldn't have them or had to deny myself. So if I was in a restaurant and they brought a bowl of sweets with the bill I would put some in my bag or pocket, I just didn't feel I had to eat them. One day I just chucked the whole lot out as they had been accumulating in the tin for so long.

I didn't ever imagine I could be indifferent to chocolate or cake. I was a true chocaholic. Once I could not even keep it in the house without eating it all, I even ate all the chocolate decorations from the Christmas tree within a day of hanging them up. At my daughter's christening when all the guests had left and we were clearing up my au pair and I decided we should immediately eat all the cakes that were left over so they were out of the way and could not tempt us. Having to eat them to be free of them meant the cakes were more powerful than me. Now I can eat chocolate but I don't need very much of it, it doesn't taste that special any more because I no longer tell myself it's special and after one or two pieces I have had enough. You will find that you can do this too, not just with chocolate but with all junk food.

Remind yourself of this fact when you come across foods you have told yourself are hard to resist:

- I will always have another day to eat this.
- It's not free and it will cost me to eat this.
- I have all my life to eat cake/pizza. Looking the way I want to look is more important right now.

When You Eat Less You Get to Eat *More*

Another way to look at it is to see that by restricting your diet you actually get to eat more. This is a long-term view, but it's important. By choosing to eat differently you will live longer and live a fuller, healthier life. A longer life means you get to eat more than if, in the short term, you eat anything and everything because you hate feeling deprived. If you enjoy eating and you want to eat a lot, think about the years ahead of you and all the opportunities you will have to eat the foods you love rather than eating them in large quantities right now. When you make these small adjustments you are not eating less and suffering more you are actually eating more in the long term and not suffering at all. You will be free of feeling hungry, deprived or different and instead of feeling that you are fighting a never-ending battle you will know that you are already winning.

This may sound extreme but it is a reality. For example, I was scheduled to see a client after he had his stomach stapled. The day before his surgery he went on a bingeing feast and died on the operating table from heart problems. If he had eaten less he would still be here. He lost his life because he believed he loved food too much to cut down and that supposed love of food cost him maybe forty years of eating since he was only forty when he died.

My favourite comedian, John Candy, died aged forty-three because of his weight problems, and my favourite singer Barry White died aged only fifty-eight due to weight-related issues. Luther Vandross died from weight problems aged fifty-four. The soul singer Rick James was being considered for *Celebrity Fit Club USA* and died only weeks before filming because of a weight-related illness.

We could have enjoyed so much more of them and they could have had a longer, fuller life if only they had taken control of their eating.

Not everyone can be naturally skinny. Some people are built bigger and will gain weight more easily, especially if they keep eating the wrong type of food. Even if that is you, you can still be a healthy weight and have a respectful, healthy and happy relationship with food. Limiting certain foods is not the same as going on a diet. You don't have to go hungry or count calories. You can eat very well and eat very healthy food while shedding weight. You simply have to choose to make other choices.

Think Thin, Get Thin

If you want to change your actions you must begin by changing your thoughts. As John Drained said, 'We first make our habits and then our habits make us.' If your habit of action is eating chocolate and your habit of thought is chocolate cheers me up and makes everything better you have to give up the thought habit as well as the action habit if you want to reach and stay at your ideal weight. Of course, thoughts don't start off as ingrained habits but once an idea has been accepted it tends to stick. The longer it is held the more it tends to become a fixed habit of thinking. Moreover, people on diets only focus on giving up the action while still believing the same thoughts, which is why they resume overeating and regain the weight. On this programme you are totally changing your thought habits, so changing your eating habits becomes a conclusion.

We have many thought habits that are incorrect but are still fixed in the mind. Some people believe that at critical times they must eat or have a drink to steady their nerves. Others believe a tranquilliser or cigarette is needed to calm them down. This is not necessarily true. The tranquilliser or drink they take could be a placebo, but the idea is there and it is a fixed habit of thought.

These are fixed ideas not fleeting thoughts, but no matter how fixed the ideas are or how long they have been held they absolutely *can* be changed. For example, in the West we believe we need lots of milk for calcium, whereas this belief does not exist in the East and people are not suffering with osteoporosis to the same degree. In fact, they have fewer bone fractures in the East than in the West. Another example is that many of us eat when we are tired because we believe the food will give us energy. However, digesting food takes up masses of energy so eating when we are tired at night is ineffective. If you come in late in the evening and are tired you don't need to eat anything. Just go to bed and save your eating until the morning. You won't get any benefit from late-night eating, the food will be much harder to digest through the night and you will wake up still feeling tired because your body has been working all night to digest food it didn't want or need.

All beliefs can be changed if you introduce doubt. The minute you begin to question something you no longer really believe it. People in lots of countries don't consume cow's milk, nor do they believe it has any benefits. Many cultures don't consume table salt or table sugar and again they don't believe they are missing any-thing. I am amazed at how many of my clients tell me, 'You need salt, it's important' or 'My body needs sugar to function', despite all the public health information initiatives over the past few years. There is so much salt in modern processed food we don't need to add more – ever. Nor do we need sugar as we get plenty of it from fruit and other foods.

Look at all your beliefs about food, your weight, your eating habits and your body. You can introduce doubt into any belief, conviction or opinion you have that is negative about your body. This is especially true if you have a belief that you cannot lose weight. If you became ill and could not eat for a while you would lose weight, so it's not physically impossible.

Run Your Brain, Reduce Your Weight

To change negative reactions in your body, i.e. overeating or continuing to eat when you are full or bingeing on chocolate, it is important to change the ideas responsible for the reaction both consciously and subconsciously. The brain and nervous system respond to mental images regardless of whether the image is self induced or from the external world. The mental image formed becomes the blueprint, and the subconscious mind uses every means at its disposal to carry out the picture. That's why cinemas show us pictures of food and drink so we'll want them. Every time you say, 'I gain weight just by looking at food' you are making your mind and body believe this thought and act upon it. Every time you say, 'My metabolism doesn't work properly' or 'I was born heavy' you are doing the same thing.

People with weight issues frequently say, 'I can't leave food', 'I can't say no to it' or 'I don't know when I have had enough, I don't know what full is.' Slim people will say the opposite: 'I can't finish it', 'I have had enough' or 'I couldn't eat another mouthful.' Just as some people eat when they are upset as they believe it will comfort them, others cannot eat when they feel upset because they don't hold that belief. You are able to choose what you say and to choose how you eat. Changing your eating habits is not enough, you must change your thoughts, beliefs and words as well.

Work through the following quick exercise to see the power of your thoughts.

As you read through these next few lines just imagine that you are standing in your kitchen and you are holding a lemon that you have just taken from the fridge. It feels cold in your hand. Look at the outside of it, the yellow waxy skin that comes to a small green point at both ends. Squeeze it a little and feel its firmness and its weight. Imagine raising the lemon to your nose and smelling that unique fresh lemon smell. Now imagine cutting the lemon in half and inhale it. The smell is stronger. Now imagine biting deeply into the lemon and letting the juice swirl around in your mouth. Taste the sharpness, the fresh citrus flavour. At this point, if you have used your imagination well, your mouth will be watering.

Consider the implications of this. Words, mere words, affected your salivary glands. The words did not even reflect reality, but something you imagined. When you read those words about the lemon you were telling your brain you had a lemon. Although you did not mean it your brain took it seriously and said to your salivary glands, 'she/he is biting a lemon, hurry, wash it away'. Your glands obeyed.

If something as simple as imagining you were eating a lemon can cause your body to react physically then something as simple as imagining you are eating selectively and shedding weight can and will cause your body to react physically too.

Words do not just reflect reality; they can create reality – like the flow of saliva you just caused by doing the exercise. The subconscious mind is no subtle interpreter of your intentions, it receives information and it stores it, it believes without question everything you tell it since its job is not to question but to act immediately on your instructions, which to your subconscious mind are commands. Tell your subconscious mind something like 'I am eating a lemon' and it goes to work. That experiment was neutral, so physically no good or harm can come from it, but good as well as harm can come from many of the words we use.

If you are on an aeroplane waiting to fly to California you may be filling your mind with images of the shopping you are going to do, the beaches you are going to visit, the weather you are going to enjoy and you will respond to those images. The person next to you may be filling their mind with images of fear. They may believe that some of the passengers look like terrorists and as they focus on the fact that the plane may crash they will respond to those images by becoming agitated and nervous. So two people on the same flight are responding differently because of the words and images they are creating.

The way we feel at any given time is due to what we focus on and what our focus comes from:

- The pictures we make in our head.
- The words we say to ourselves.

The good news is that we can change those words and pictures at any time and we can learn to make them more positive all the time.

Scientists and doctors have noted that patients respond very well to positive suggestions. They reason that each of us has two selves – a conscious and a subconscious self. The conscious self that you are aware of has an unreliable memory, whereas the subconscious self has an amazing memory. It registers without our knowledge the smallest events and it accepts without reasoning whatever we tell it.

If your subconscious believes that your metabolic system is functioning successfully then it will. However, if it has accepted a suggestion that you come from a fat family and are helpless to do anything about it, then notwithstanding the fact that you were born with a normal weight and metabolism you are much more likely to remain overweight.

These suggestions caused by negative beliefs, which you may not be consciously aware of, form blocks in your mind. By changing your belief system as you work your way through this book and repeating your new affirmations, as well as playing your audio download, you can and will overcome them.

Our subconscious presides over all our actions, whatever they are. This is what we call imagination; contrary to accepted opinion, imagination always makes us act, even against our will. It is a rule of the mind that your imagination always beats your willpower, in a battle between willpower and imagination the imagination will always win without exception. One of the rules of the mind is that imagination is far more powerful than knowledge and that emotion is more powerful than logic when dealing with our own minds and those of other people. For example, if I asked you to stand on a small narrow coffee table you could do it easily. If I asked you to walk a plank of wood placed a few inches off the ground, you would walk along it effortlessly because you would imagine it to be easy. You would see yourself walking across without difficulty. Now, I want you to imagine walking that same plank of wood while it is placed between two very high buildings, within two steps you would begin to tremble and you would be very likely to fall off. Imagine the coffee table is now the window ledge on the top floor of a sky scraper; can you stand on it easily? You could stand on that amount of space when it was a table because your imagination told you it was okay. Now your imagination is telling you that you could fall, you could die, this is dangerous and crazy and your same imagination will stop you doing it.

So why is it that you would not fall off the plank nearer the ground? When the plank was on the ground you believed that you could do it. When the plank was placed between the high buildings you imagined that you could not do it, even if you were offered a lot of money, because your imagination sees you falling. In the scenario with the high buildings your will is powerless against your imagination. If you have been on many diets and had no long-term success your imagination will now see any diet failing to work for you. It is the rule of the mind that your imagination will always win.

The aim of my programme is to train your imagination so that you will win. Your imagination is like an untamed horse, it is immensely powerful but you have to train it to go where you want it to go. Your imagination and your ability to see yourself as slimmer, to believe you can become and stay a lighter weight and to be indifferent to food is more powerful than any outdated data that says it can't be done. Modern science has now proven that the way you think can physically change your body. Changing your thinking can and does change your body.

The Power of Your Mind

I know you don't just want to hear this, to believe it you need to see it and experience it for yourself. The following test will do that for you. Many of my clients find this very useful because it gives them absolute proof that our thoughts affect our bodies. Once you have that proof you can never again say, 'I can't help it, it's just the way I am'. The truth is it's the way you think not the way you are and the following test will really change your thinking which in turn will change your body.

You need someone to help you do this. First, make a fist and make one arm as strong and rigid as you can. Hold that arm out in front of you at shoulder height and get your helper to push down on that arm to test your strength, while you use all your strength to resist them. Now you have established your strength think of the most negative words or beliefs you use about yourself in relation to your weight and how you eat. Repeat these words out loud ten times or just think them silently, ten times, for example, 'I am fat' or 'I can't lose weight' or 'I can't stop eating'. Now thinking these thoughts make your arm strong again and repeat the strength testing process. Have someone push down on your rigid arm, you will find that as you think negative thoughts you lose your strength and your arm can easily be pushed down. Amazing isn't it? When you think those negative thoughts you are losing all the strength in your muscles and your arm is becoming weak.

Now think of some positive thoughts repeat them silently or out loud ten times, for example, 'I am shedding weight and loving the process' or 'I have a totally different attitude to food now and always', or 'I will stay at my ideal weight'.

Now thinking these thoughts make your arm strong again and repeat the strength testing process. As you think positive thoughts you become physically stronger, it will be easier for you to resist the pushing on your arm. Every thought you have creates a physical reaction in the body and you have just proved it to yourself.

Where a thought goes, energy goes with it, so changing your thinking and using different language really can change your body. Most people are fascinated by this testing, and since it's such an interesting process I recommend you spend some time experimenting with it:

1 Repeating all the negative thoughts and beliefs you had.
2 Using all the negative words you had been using before realising the power of language.
3 Testing your strength.
4 Replacing these negative beliefs with positive constructive beliefs.
5 Testing your strength again and seeing the difference.

You can do this with so many beliefs, not only in the area of weight and addictions but in beliefs you have about your confidence, self esteem, habits, abilities, relationships, in fact anything at all.

Remember, these beliefs only exist in your imagination and you are free to change your thinking and your language as soon as you become aware of how limiting and destructive your language and beliefs are.

- **Your thoughts are yours to change.**
- **Your mind is yours to direct.**
- **Your body shape and eating habits are absolutely yours to change.**

Visualisation to Keep You Thinner

In order to be slim you absolutely *must* be able to see yourself as slim. This is not natural or easy for someone who has been over-weight for a long time but you can do it with practice. Just taking five minutes a day, every day, to visualise yourself as slim, with a selective attitude to food, will work.

Scientists in many countries have now absolutely proved that visualisation skills significantly improve weight loss and its maintenance. When you see yourself as thin you send a clear message to your mind that influences your energy, your metabolism, your appetite and your attitude towards your body. These changes have a positive impact on your thoughts and feelings, which in turn reinforce the mind conditioning and your motivation.

How does it actually work? Well, thinking positively about weight reduction can activate particular neurons in the brain; these neurons can secrete hormones such as endogenous opiates which make us feel good about ourselves and allow us to stop comfort eating. Negative thoughts have the opposite effect: particular neurons are involved with producing a negative thought and they also produce negative hormones such as cortisol, which is a stress hormone, and stress leads to comfort eating and overeating. Stress leads to over-production of cortisol; cortisol aids addictive behaviour and encourages us to overeat on junk food.

Remember, habits are merely thoughts and actions that we have learned and practised, we are not born craving sugar or eating crisps when we are stressed, we learned to overeat or binge on these foods to give us a feeling of comfort. When you repeat an action you create a neural pathway to your brain that is strengthened with each repetition. This pathway is like a thread that becomes stronger every time you repeat something. When you first learned to use a computer, drive a car or operate a new mobile phone or any kind of machinery you had to repeat the actions slowly, but now, due to repetition, they are so embedded in you they are almost automatic.

When we cease the habit the pathways diminish and become redundant. I call this rewiring ourselves. We come into the world wired for success and this programme is putting the wiring back as it should be so that you can have a normal relationship with food and your body.

So the key is repetition of these positive visualisations. It takes repeating and practising something twenty-one times over twenty-one days for the brain to create new neurological habit pathways, and in turn it takes twenty-one days for those pathways to begin to diminish if you cease the actions. Various studies have shown that it takes the brain a minimum of ten days and a maximum of twenty-one days to let go of an old belief and replace it with another one. Twenty-one days of affirmations and new habits of language and beliefs will start to lock in good and positive changes for you. After twenty-one days you will also have different blood sugar and be losing the old sugar and junk food cravings. You need to continue the affirmations but eventually this will cease being what you do and become who you are, so it will be automatic. Remember you will have your audio download to use to help you even more.

Becoming skilled and adept at visualisation requires you to focus on your new positive images frequently and to use repetition until it is so easy it becomes automatic. Repetition is vital, and the more vividly you visualise the more rapidly your mind and body responds. This is exactly what you do when you drive a car or operate machinery – you visualise the actions you have to take, then take them until the process becomes almost automatic.

Every time you visualise:

- Make the picture exciting and compelling.
- Increase the duration and intensity.
- Hold the picture for longer.
- Make it bigger, brighter and clearer.
- Add exciting positive words.

Combining visualisation images with intensity of desire while telling yourself you are succeeding will increase the effectiveness.

Visualisation takes practice but remind yourself that what the subconscious sees it accepts. Your ability to visualise will have a powerful effect on you and as you visualise you will stimulate your mind and body into action. Remember, what you can hold in your mind with confidence you can achieve – athletes who visualise can stimulate all their muscles to perform at a level to meet their visualisation. Become more clear and detailed about what you want. The more you visualise the more you will believe your visualisation is possible.

Lots of very successful people visualise all the time. Great actors are by nature very visual; just as they can see themselves playing a psycho or heroine and pull it off, they can see themselves as being slim (if it's important to them or the part they are playing) and successful and this becomes the image they hold in their mind and move towards.

We can all change our thinking and the mental pictures we make and as we improve them we improve everything. By changing your thinking and your focus and by making changes to the pictures you form in your mind and the language you use, you can change your body, your weight and your life.

If you think you can't visualise, then you need to be aware that you are already visualising all the time. Every time you say, 'I can't leave chips', 'It's impossible for me to refuse cake', 'If I go there I know I will overeat', 'I can't lose weight', 'I can't keep the weight off', 'If I look at food I get fat', 'If I eat one I can't stop', 'Biscuits are my downfall', 'Crisps are my weakness', you are already visualising negatively and it's working, but not to your advantage! You might as well use good visualisations as your mind will believe and act upon whatever you tell it, good or bad. You have nothing to lose (apart from excess body fat) and everything to gain (apart from weight) by making the words and pictures positive.

Occasionally I come across clients who say to me, 'I am just not visual and I can't visualise at all'. Sometimes I tease them a bit by saying, 'Lucky you, that's amazing, you must never have a day's worry in your life.' When they reply, 'Are you kidding? I worry about everything: my kids, my job, my health.' I then ask them, 'But how can you worry if you can't visualise? that's what worry is – visualising what could go wrong.' We are all visual, some of us just don't know how visual we are – but you do now.

You would never find your car in a car park if, on your return, you didn't visualise where you had put it. When you go to a supermarket it's your visualisation skills that take you to familiar aisles on auto pilot. When you learn to cook a particular dish, you refer to the recipe but if you cook it a lot the process will become so visual you will easily prepare it without referring to the recipe at all. If I ask you to describe the layout of your bedroom, the colour of the sheets and what's on your bedside table, you first have to visualise – mentally imagine how they look by picturing them. We can all do this.

Many people visualise getting the weight off and stop there, they don't make it a lifetime picture and instead they often picture how hard it is going to be to maintain their new reduced weight. While you are visualising becoming slimmer, visualise it as a way of life and see yourself staying at your ideal weight. Many people have kept off their previous excess weight, including Oprah Winfrey, Sarah Ferguson, Nigel Lawson, Jennifer Aniston, Belinda Carlisle and Sophie Dahl and they are not suffering deprivation. You can do the very same thing.

I had a battle to be slim for years to such an extent that it almost ruled my life and I couldn't imagine not having it. Now I have been free of it for so long and I know it will never come back. My body is used to how I eat now and used to the weight I am and it will stay like that.

It's not a good idea to keep your fat clothes just in case, what kind of message are you sending to yourself when you do that? It's not a good idea to keep buying clothes that are bigger than you need because you don't have faith that you will keep the weight off. Have faith, conviction and unshakable certainty that you will and you are constantly succeeding and it will happen.

This is to show you the effect visualising has on your body:

1 Stand up, take one arm, raise it to shoulder height and, pointing your finger directly out in front of you, begin to turn your arm as far out and behind you as you can. If it's your right arm move it out to the right, if it's your left move it out to the left. When you have moved your arm as far behind you as you can, look behind you and notice where it is.

2 Now return your arm to the starting position in front of you then close your eyes for a moment. Just imagine and see your arm moving even further, up to 25 per cent further behind you, really see this in your mind for a moment. Now tell yourself your arm is going to move 25 per cent further. Say this to yourself three or four times.

3 Now open your eyes repeat the arm movement and notice just how much further your arm will go.

You are already beginning to see the power of beliefs on the body. As you saw, believed and thought about your arm moving further, it did. Do it a few more times to prove to yourself how easy it is to influence your body using your belief system. Athletes have been using this technique for years – seeing themselves lifting a heavier weight or performing a longer jump, believing they will do it and can do it and then doing exactly that. In fact, many tests have been undertaken proving that in athletics the ability to visualise is equally as important as physical training. When an athlete visualises they can cause all their muscles to perform at a level to meet the visualisation. It is now becoming accepted that in the future it is likely that only athletes who use powers of visualisation, as well as training, will succeed because they have an edge and advantage over others.

I recently made a television documentary with some of my clients who are Olympic athletes. They were talking about how many athletes from many different countries at the last Olympic Games used the power of thought, belief and visualisation to succeed and how it gave them an advantage over those who didn't and helped them break a world record.

You may have heard stories of people who are slightly built or unfit lifting a heavy object like a car, tree or refrigerator off their child who was trapped underneath, and then wondering how they managed it. In fact, they momentarily saw themselves performing the feat and then performed it because their mind, in that moment, believed they could and would do it. You are now ready to believe you can and will reach and maintain your ideal weight and that you will do what it takes happily and willingly and that your body is responding to your new and good visualisations.

Visualisation is not just about what you see, it's also about what you feel and hear and say. It makes your visualisation more powerful when you activate all your senses as you visualise. The more senses you activate the more real your feeling is that you will and are already accomplishing this so while you are visualising be sure to:

- *Feel* that there is less of you when you are showering.
- *Feel* your waistband becoming looser when you dress.
- *Hear* people tell you how much slimmer you look.
- *Hear* all the praise and compliments coming your way.
- *Hear* the shop assistant telling you that you need a smaller size.
- *See* yourself buying clothes in a smaller size and throwing out your fat clothes.
- *See* yourself shunning junk food.
- *Sense* how very well you are doing.
- *Sense* how strong and committed to change you are.
- *Sense* your taste buds are changing as you like healthy food now.

At the same time as forming different pictures in your mind you must tell yourself different things. Eliminate every possible negative word, focus only on what you wish to achieve and move towards. Keep your mind on what you want and off what you don't want. Whatever you focus on you will move towards, so thinking about how you don't want to look and what you don't want to eat simply puts negative words and images back into your mind. Tell yourself, 'I feel full and satisfied', not 'I am not so hungry anymore'. Think, 'I am reducing weight easily and enjoying the process', or 'I prefer my new food choices. I like this way of eating it works for me' rather than 'I no longer feel fat. I don't want to eat chocolate anymore.' Visualise, think and say, 'My body is leaner and healthier' not 'I don't look as overweight'. Focus your thoughts positively, 'I feel so committed to this programme, it feels so right' not 'It's not as hard as I thought it would be'.

'No', 'not' and 'don't' are all neutral words in that they don't make a picture and have little effect on the subconscious mind. Thinking I am *not* hungry, I *don't* crave chocolate, I *don't* want to eat chips, causes the mind to lock onto the only descriptive words in the sentence – *hungry*, *chips* and *chocolate*.

If I ask you not to think of pink snow in order not to think of it you have to think of it and see it even though you have never seen pink snow before. Try right now not to think of pink snow and you will see what happens – you cannot help thinking about it. By turning over any negative thoughts you will find the positive. The subconscious mind is only in the moment; therefore when you visualise create images that are occurring now, this instant. For example, 'My body is becoming more fit, healthy and attractive every day', or 'I am adapting to this new eating lifestyle so well and dropping weight'.

Make your words dynamic and descriptive: 'I am confident and so successful with my diet'.

Make it personal:

- *I am slimmer.*
- *I look leaner.*
- *I will make it work.*
- *I always make healthy food choices.*
- *I can do this, I enjoy it.*
- *I do whatever it takes willingly.*
- *I always eat this way now and it always works.*

Using the 'I am, I can' technique, add your own words to the statement below or make a completely unique one incorporating changes that are personal to your own life so your statement reads something like this:

I feel so confident about my body, I am slimmer and becoming leaner and lighter all the time. I feel proud when I look at the contents of my shopping basket; I always make healthy food choices. It feels great when people pay me compliments. Knowing I will reach my ideal weight, I am taking control of my life. I look so much slimmer and feel happy. I will eat this way for the rest of my life. I willingly and happily do whatever it takes. I love going to the gym and always make time to exercise. I always have portable food to hand. I am wearing smaller clothes. I look good, I feel amazing, my body loves what I am doing for it. I am in great shape physically and mentally and my healthy attitude to food and my body keeps me slim.

You can add things like, 'My partner admires me', 'I go swimming with my children', 'I wear ————', 'I look and feel younger'. Whatever is appropriate and inspiring for you. Write it out and put it somewhere you can read it every day.

Visualise Your Progress

Many people get disheartened on diets. They may drop a lot of weight quickly and then put it all back on again. As a result people shed the same 10 pounds over and over again. It is better to shed weight realistically. Two pounds a week is a great achievement, if you get to a point where you feel disheartened because you have only shed 5 pounds, carry around a 5 pound chicken or 5 pounds of potatoes all day or even for twenty minutes and you will soon feel very different and pleased that you have shed all that weight and be inspired to shed more. I was explaining this to the participants on *Celebrity Fit Club USA* and the following week the host mentioned that he had being doing that all week, carrying around an item that weighed 5 pounds for a few hours each day and it had totally changed his attitude and left him proud of the weight he'd shed and excited and inspired to shed more. Instead of feeling that he was not making enough progress he could literally feel the amount of weight he had already shed and it motivated him to continue.

Next time you are in a supermarket pick up an item equivalent to the weight you have shed – it can be anything from a bag of soap powder to a turkey to a bag of carrots. If you want to be precise you can even weigh out some carrots to the exact amount of weight you have reduced by. Carry that item around the shop in your hand not in the trolley and feel how heavy it is. Then feel so good about dropping that amount of weight and excited by your progress and inspired to make even more.

Breaking Patterns

To find the most effective way of breaking the patterns that you have picked up through your life in relation to overeating, take the following test to see which type of eater you are and therefore which methods are best suited to getting results.

There are six types of overeater and they are:

- Addictive eaters.
- Emotional eaters.
- Habitual eaters.
- Ignorant eaters.
- Destructive eaters.
- Angry eaters.

Answer the following questions to find out which one you are or are predominantly. If you answer yes to more than 50 per cent of the questions you can identify yourself with that category.

- Do you think about food all day then, when you are eating, cram food into your mouth and eat really fast so you don't even taste it and want more food?
- Do you repeat this pattern over and over?

- Do you crave sugar? If you have sugary snacks in the house do you eat them and are unable to save them for later or another day?
- Do you eat sensibly all day and only break your diet in the evenings?
- Are there some foods that once you start eating them you can't stop? i.e. jumbo bags of crisps or family size bars of chocolate?
- Do you eat something like a bar of chocolate so fast that when it's finished you realise you didn't enjoy it, savour it or really even taste it?

If you have answered yes, you are an addictive eater.

- Do you overeat in secret?
- Do you use food to block your emotions and feelings, i.e. eating when you are lonely, unhappy or bored?
- Do you prefer to eat alone and do you eat differently when eating with others?
- Would you find it hard to be without chocolate, sweets and biscuits?
- Do you at times crave food full of salt, fat or sugar?
- Do you eat when under pressure?
- Do you particularly crave carbohydrates when you are unhappy?
- Do you believe that certain foods comfort you and make you feel better?

If you have answered yes, you are an emotional eater.

- Are your children or partner overweight?
- Do you no longer recognise when you are full and when you are hungry?
- Do you put on weight predominantly around your stomach?
- Do you eat whenever food is in front of you regardless of whether or not you are hungry?

- Do you finish everything and always clear your plate?
- Do you find it particularly hard to throw food away or 'waste' it?
- Were you always made to finish meals as a child?
- Do you find yourself using every occasion to eat i.e. watching television, in a car or on a train journey, at the cinema, etc?
- Do you eat quickly and finish before others?

If you have answered yes, you are a habitual eater.

- Do you think that all salad is healthy including coleslaw and the dressing?
- Do you think cheese is good for you and pizza is a complete meal because it has some peppers and tomatoes on it?
- Do you believe that bread, potatoes, cereal and milk are good foods?
- Do you think all foods labelled low fat, reduced sugar and diet must be good for you?
- Do you count potatoes as vegetables?
- Do you think fruit bars, fruit drinks and canned fruit are as good as fresh fruit?

If you have answered yes, you are an ignorant eater.

- Do you sabotage your diet every time you come close to your ideal weight?
- Do you feel anxious and uncomfortable when you are slimmer?
- Do you still buy clothes in bigger sizes and keep your fat clothes?
- Do you shed the same 10 pounds (or thereabouts) every year then gain it back?
- Do you feel more comfortable when your body is covered up and uneasy when it is on show, i.e. do you prefer winter because you can wear layers and hate summer because you are supposed to wear less?

- Do you celebrate your weight loss success by resuming eating the foods you had denied yourself?

If you have answered yes, you are a destructive eater.

- Do you prefer crunchy food like crisps, nachos, apples, popcorn, French bread or very chewy food like toffee and beef jerky?
- Do you feel better after chewing and biting food?
- Do you eat something after an argument or if you feel tense or wound up because it changes your state?
- Do you feel agitated if you have to wait too long for your food to be served to you in a restaurant or on an airline?

If you have answered yes, you are an angry eater.

It's Not What You're Eating It's What's Eating You

Addictive eaters crave sugary food, caffeine, junk food, colas and refined carbohydrates because they are addicted to the chemical composition of these foods. They always find these foods stimulate them to want more and have great difficulty resisting them or eating just a little of this type of food. The pleasure centre of the brain releases dopamine when we eat chemicals, fat and sugar, dopamine gives us the same high that drugs and alcohol do.

Emotional eaters find loneliness, boredom and sadness are temporarily abated when they fill their stomachs with refined carbohydrates. They fill them up quickly and they feel satisfied and sedated, even tranquillised, for a while. Comfort can briefly be found in soft sweet foods like ice cream or cake that reminds us of childhood. Depressed people often want caffeine and sugary foods. Emotional eaters try to get rid of a bad feeling fast and try to feel good even faster by using comfort foods and bulk eating.

Habitual eaters have often been made to eat everything on their plate. As children they were often not allowed to leave food and have conditioned themselves to continue this habit. They will eat at every occasion and eat everything in front of them without being aware of whether they are hungry or not.

Ignorant eaters have been completely brainwashed by food manufacturers to believe that what they are eating is healthy or harmless. They eat a lot of convenience and ready meals and believe they are as good as home-cooked food. They may exist primarily on diet foods and diet drinks but still have a weight problem.

Destructive eaters usually have a deep-rooted need to hide their sexuality and feel vulnerable when they look attractive or desirable. People who have never had enough like volume and frequency of meals as they always feel they may not get enough. They often feel panicky in a situation where food is shared, i.e. a group Chinese meal, in case they get less. They feel uncomfortable when they cannot dish out their own portions and a host does it for them in case they don't get enough to satisfy them.

Angry eaters like crunchy food like crisps and apples and tough food like meat and thick bread that they can chomp and chew on. Hard mastication is effective when we are feeling tense and wound up. Stressed people often want salty foods. They will always eat after a fight or disagreement to make themselves feel better.

As you categorise which type of eater you are you can use the following case histories to find the right affirmations to change your habits of thought and actions. If you fall into more than one category that is okay and not unusual, just use the affirmations for both categories. People of a normal weight will answer yes to some of the questions – the difference is it does not run their lives. It might help you to know that over 70 per cent of over-eaters are emotional eaters and addictive eaters. Another 20 per cent are habitual and ignorant eaters. Only around 10 per cent fall into the destructive and the angry category.

Up to 43 per cent of people use food to alter their moods every single day. There is so much going on behind our seemingly unconscious eating habits. It is essential that you know what your issues are in order to fix them because it's hard to fix what you don't understand, but once you have that understanding you also have the power to change. The understanding and the solutions that each chapter offers you are changing you on every level. In the next chapter you will find the information to adjust how you eat. These adjustments are crucial for addictive eaters.

As you read some of my client case histories you may find one or more that feel applicable to you or that resonate with you. If so follow the instructions for that person in order to sever the emotional links that have caused you to eat badly (or incorrectly). Of course you may need to alter the affirmations since we are all unique and following the case histories you will find instructions telling you exactly how to do that.

For many overweight people the weight is simply the presenting problem – the visible effect or symptom of the real problem underneath. Excess weight can have a role, a function and a purpose. Often it is to insulate someone from being rejected or to hide their sexuality from the world or to offer up as a reason for failure: 'I could have been a success if only I was thinner', 'He/she would have liked me if I was not overweight', or 'I would have got that job if I wasn't so fat', and so on. Once the true reason for the excess weight is uncovered most clients go on to reduce their weight and keep it off permanently.

Addictive Eaters

Lorna had battled with her weight for years. She was a compulsive eater and craved food almost all the time. She told me that she had begun to develop very early and had noticeable breasts when she was ten. Her mother was horrified by this and put her on a very restrictive diet to stop her body developing. Lorna did not want to be denied food and resisted all her mother's attempts to put her on the grapefruit diet or any kind of diet. While her family were having toast and cereal for breakfast she was given only half a grapefruit. Soon Lorna was banned from eating any kind of cakes, biscuits, desserts or bread although other family members ate them freely and in her presence. Her mother was so determined to make Lorna thinner that she locked the pantry and put her on a 1,000 calorie a day diet. Lorna told me she would volunteer to clear the table and wash up just so she could secretly eat the rest of her family's leftovers. She would wolf down food from anybody's plate rather than be denied it. Because she was deprived of food and had no say in the matter, while her friends and family were allowed to eat with no restriction, she developed an obsession with the very food she had been denied: sugar, junk food and refined carbs. She ate them so often, in an outdated need to defy her mother and take back control, she had become addicted to them. We cured the addiction once she understood how and why it had begun.

Solution

The following statements are essential to changing your addiction habits. Remember the explanation I've previously given of how they work and use them to work for you:

- I can have whatever I want now but I just don't need it.
- I am choosing to be slim and healthy for me not anyone else because I can, I am ready, I want to and it's easy now.
- My understanding gives me power and freedom to be the correct weight for me.
- I recognise addictive foods and happily refuse them.
- Sugar is not a food. I enjoy its absence and feel better without it than I ever thought I did with it.

Like Lorna, Barbara had a very controlling mother. She was not put on a diet but she was not allowed any kind of sweets or biscuits. Her mother very strictly enforced this; at school if the children brought in a birthday cake to share she was not allowed any of it. At birthday parties she was not allowed any of the cakes or chocolate. Her mother could only enforce this when Barbara was small but even in her teens no sugar was allowed in the house. As soon as Barbara had her own money she would buy as much confectionery as she could afford and eat it all at once setting up a long-lasting sugar addiction. She was very overweight but could not stay on any diet as the foods they forbade were the very same foods her mother banned (sweets, biscuits and cake) and she linked pain to being denied them and pleasure to eating them. Diets tell you what you can't have, many people have a desire to eat the very foods they are forbidden. It is human nature to want the things we are denied, hence people on Atkins who crave fruit when they did not even want it much beforehand. You can only stop eating certain foods by choosing to, not by being made to.

Solution

Use the following statements to give your body the messages you want it to respond to:

- I am choosing to eat like an adult, to eat the foods that are right for me.
- I love the feeling that I am in control now.
- Everything is available to me now, including being my ideal weight.
- I can and do choose what to eat and what I weigh.
- I could have junk food but I am choosing not to.
- Instead I choose to be slim.
- My mother is not in control, I am and I willingly make the right choices for me.
- Biscuits are for babies.
- Cakes are for children.

Emotional Eaters

Amy was an emotional eater who had an addiction to cakes and biscuits and ate them daily. She ate them even more when she was unhappy, sad or bored. Her mother worked away a lot and didn't spend much time with Amy. On special events like birthdays she would put a lot of time and effort into making Amy a cake and this made Amy feel special. It seemed that Amy tried to get that special feeling back by eating the same food her mother had made her. Since her mother's death Amy had only wanted to eat cakes. If our mothers make us rice pudding with strawberry jam or apple pie when we are unhappy we often want those very same foods whenever we feel low. Again part of breaking the pattern is to fully understand how we acquired it in the first place since we all come into the world with normal eating habits. Understanding why can be a powerful tool in letting go, as you can't change what you don't understand. When we say, 'I don't know why I do this (eat like this) I just can't seem to help it', we are taking no responsibility. Once you can say, 'I understand exactly why I did this and I choose not to do it any longer', you are taking control and becoming free. Like Amy, it is normal to cross over into more than one category.

Solution
Adapt the following suggestions to suit you, substituting your specific food, i.e. chocolate, biscuits, pizza, ice cream, fast food, in place of cake:

- Cakes aren't special, I am special.
- I understand why I thought cakes were love and accept that they never have been or could be.
- I don't need food to recreate a memory. I use my brilliant brain to do that.
- Now that I accept that I am special I eat food that makes me feel good physically and emotionally: natural food that nourishes me and keeps me slim.

Patrick was a very successful city trader who would begin each day eating normally but after a business lunch he would send his secretary out to buy him a box of cream cakes. He would eat them all then feel disgusted with himself. Every day he vowed not to eat cream cakes but on the days when he did avoid them he would stand at his fridge door in the middle of the night eating cream and chocolate instead.

In hypnosis Patrick remembered being poor during the 1960s and only having the most basic food to eat. He and his friends would walk to school and on the way they would stop to look into the window of a nearby bakery. Patrick would look at all the fancy cakes and say out loud, 'When I grow up I am going to eat all of these every day'. He and his friends would amuse themselves by picking out the cakes that they would enjoy the most if only they could afford to buy them saying to each other, 'I will have that one first, then that one, then that one', in doing so they could forget that they were dirt poor for a few moments. Patrick told me this was a ritual that he indulged in every morning and afternoon for years on his way past the bakery. His brain clearly got the message and acted on it because years later he was doing just what he had visualised, eating cakes and chocolate excessively.

If as a child you long for a certain type of food and link enormous pleasure to eating it in abundance, if you frequently focus on that longing and repeat it regularly, then your mind will assume you want that and the emotional imprint will be far stronger than the logic that tries to ignore it or fight it.

Patrick was wealthy, successful and heading for a heart attack as his cholesterol level was alarmingly high. He understood in hypnosis that he was acting from an outdated and redundant longing and that in his mind he had linked being successful with eating high-calorie confectionery. By having Patrick state over and over again, 'I am forty-five, I have money, I can have cakes every day but I choose not to, I'm free of them', he was able to lose all interest in them.

Solution

Do exactly the same if you have a history of not being allowed certain foods as a child and longed for them. Many children were not allowed fizzy drinks and as adults they crave them for the wrong reasons. (Including me – I only got them at my grandmothers and they were an enormous treat that I continued to treat myself to as an adult. I only stopped when I was pregnant and they made me so sick I have never drunk them since.)

Repeat:

- I am an adult with freedom to choose.
- I can eat————every day but I am choosing not to.
- I am indifferent to them forever.
- I have power over those foods and they have nothing over me.
- I have money to buy the foods I want.
- I choose sophisticated grown-up food.

Martina was fourteen and obese. When I began to talk to her she told me that she was very unhappy because she felt no one took any notice of her at home. She told me that she had a much smaller bedroom than her older brother and sister and that her mother called her 'my baby' while her father called her 'my little girl'. For her parents this may have been a loving gesture but Martina felt so insignificant and so small that I wondered if she had an unconscious need to be big, to be noticed, to stand out and be a physically bigger and more important presence in her family.

To her parents' credit they came to a session and both agreed to stop referring to her to as 'my baby' and 'my little girl'. Her father moved his office into Martina's small bedroom and Martina made her father's office into a bigger bedroom. Once Martina stopped feeling so small and unimportant in her own home her weight changed, she found it easier to eat differently and she dropped two stone.

Solution

If you feel in any way insignificant or unimportant and you are overweight you must deal with the feelings of insignificance and counteract them. They are as important as the excess weight. You cannot fix one without the other because they will be interlinked. You must say:

- I am enough.
- I am significant.
- I am worth it.
- I matter.
- I am important to life.

Repeat until it is an absolute statement of truth for you and you can feel it ringing true.

Once I heard Sandra's history I told her she should never go on a deprivation or restrictive diet ever again. Sandra, who was in her sixties, told me that she would try to diet by eating as little as possible during the day. She even tried to fast or just eat fruit but by 4 o'clock she would have such an overwhelming urge to eat that she would hurry to the nearest shop and start cramming food into her mouth before she even got to the check out. She usually crammed in any kind of bread or cake and did not care what she looked like or who saw her.

In hypnosis she described living in Holland in hiding during the war and having so little food that her family once ate tulip bulbs and pet food just to have something in their stomachs. Sandra's brain had linked the most overwhelming pain to having an empty stomach. For her, going without food triggered memories of intense pain and deprivation. Her brain was so keen to move her away from this pain that it motivated her to get any food into her body as soon as possible. Our brain's job is to move us away from pain and towards pleasure.

Sandra could not diet. She could only succeed in changing what and how she ate. Although Sandra was an extreme case, denying food to someone who has been deprived of it cannot ever work. If you have ever been deprived of food because of financial circumstances or because you had a rigid controlling parent like Lorna or Barbara, any time you put yourself on a restrictive diet the memories will at some level motivate you to sabotage it. You can counteract this by telling yourself you have chosen to eat differently but do not say, 'I can't have that, I must not eat that, I am not allowed to eat those' – it just will not work long term.

Solution
Use the following affirmations to keep your eating habits in line:

- There are no restrictions.
- Only freedom of choice and free will.

- I am succeeding in changing how and what I eat forever.
- I am choosing to eat food that keeps me slim because I want to and I like it.
- I don't need to be denied anything, including the correct weight for me and I willingly adjust my eating to make this happen.

Habitual Eaters

Liam was brought up the youngest of eight brothers and sisters. Food was put on the table and the children grabbed what they could and ate as quickly as they could to stop someone else taking more than their share. If ever there were seconds the one who finished first got them. Because Liam was the smallest his elder siblings often took his food as he was too little to fight back. As a result Liam became an adult who rushed through his food and always ate as if it might run out or be taken away from him. He did not take any pleasure from eating slowly and enjoying his meals. He told me that at the table he put his head over his plate of food and literally did not raise it again until he had eaten everything in front of him. Remembering in hypnosis that he acquired these habits and came into the world with a normal attitude to food allowed him to regain the normal eating habits he was born with. He reinforced this by playing a hypnosis tape daily for three weeks and began to eat normally and regain a normal body weight.

Solution

Adapt the following statements to the particular circumstances of your own life:

- I am not eight years old, fighting for food. That's not me and never will be again.
- I am a grown-up choosing how to eat.
- I can have whatever I want whenever I want.
- I get pleasure from eating slowly savouring the taste and texture.
- I am calm and relaxed around all food.
- I love and take pleasure in leaving food. It makes me feel powerful and proves I am free from the past.
- I love eating with friends in a group. I get nourished by the conversation and atmosphere, they give me much more than food ever could.
- I interact with food, eating calmly and getting pleasure from that.

Ignorant Eaters

Ian could not understand why he was overweight as he thought he was doing everything right. He ate cereal and toast for breakfast, sandwiches for lunch, and a low-calorie ready meal or pasta and low-fat cheese in the evenings. He snacked on crackers or low-fat crisps. If he went to a fast food restaurant he ate the salad and dressing rather than burgers and fries. He always bought low-fat and reduced-fat food and drank four or five cans of diet fizzy drink a day. He was baffled about why he was overweight. I work with clients like Ian all the time and you will find all the solutions for this type of eater in the section in the next chapter called How to Eat.

Destructive Eaters

Over twenty years ago when I had just established a practice I worked with a young girl who had just landed a job as a catalogue model. Irene was very pretty and it was her dream to be a model but she was a little overweight (this was long before models looked skeletal and unhealthy) and needed to lose 10 pounds for the job. She was sent to a dietician and trainer and she lost the weight but her contract stipulated that she had to keep it off. During the fitting period in preparation for the shoot she gained it all back. She then paid for herself to go to a health farm and returned 10 pounds lighter then regained the weight even more rapidly. After this happened a third time she was sent to me and during hypnosis we uncovered in Irene an enormous fear of failure. She was so worried about not being good enough, about failing in the eyes of the public that it had become easier for her to opt out and use her weight as an excuse. In her mind it was less painful to say, 'I could have made it as a model but my weight problem stopped me', than to say, 'I got some work but I wasn't good enough to make it long term'.

Many of us fear failing and need something to blame, something that almost gives us permission to hold back, such as being overweight.

Solution
If this could be you, take a few minutes to write out how you are sabotaging yourself with weight and why it must stop and stop now. Remember to use the correct terms for your brain – do not call it fat, call it insulation or cocooning until you fully understand its purpose, its role, intention and function and can let it go.

Tanya was one of my favourite clients. She told me that she longed to be slim and had frequently lost weight on different diets. However, when she was slimmer she felt incredibly vulnerable and had a powerful urge to overeat which she always gave in to. She always gained all the weight back that she had worked hard to lose. In hypnosis Tanya regressed back to being two years old and watching from the stairs as her father hit her mother. Tanya tried to intervene and stop him but he tossed her aside like a rag doll. She reported other instances in her childhood where her father hit her mother in her presence. Tanya felt so small and vulnerable; she wanted to protect her mother but could do nothing as she was too little. These events led to Tanya feeling vulnerable when she was lighter and more secure yet unhappy when she was heavy.

Talking through this with Tanya gave her the power to move away from acting and reacting like a helpless child. It also stopped her feeling so powerless when she was lighter.

I gave her a tape to listen to every day that told her she would be slim and strong and that she had all the adult power she needed to protect herself. She had a voice and rationality and intellect and an awareness of her rights that she didn't have as a child and therefore the need to be bigger was redundant. She reached her ideal weight within four months and had kept it off for several years before we lost touch.

Solution

If you have ever felt helpless and small because you were bullied or intimidated when little and are now overweight say the same things to yourself:

- I am slender and strong.
- I am reaching my ideal weight and maintaining it while feeling safe and secure.
- I have a strong voice and I am smart. The need to be physically big is over.

Find words that work for you and repeat them every day. If you have had these issues for years it is unrealistic to expect that a week of new affirmations will give you immediate results. They could, but you also may have to repeat your new words hourly, daily and weekly to replace the years of negative conditioning.

David was obese and his story was heartbreaking. In hypnosis he regressed back to being molested frequently by a neighbour. While he was talking as if he was still that small child he kept saying, 'If only I was big these bad things would not happen to me'. Because he was so small for his age he also got bullied and beaten a lot by older children and repeated the same wish to himself, 'If I was big people couldn't hurt me'. I asked him how often he longed to be big when he was a child and he replied, 'Every hour of every day and for years'. I have seen this so often with my clients, many recall being children who were too small to protect themselves against bullying parents or siblings, or to protect their siblings or a parent from a bully. Children who are abused or molested and feel too tiny to protect themselves want to be big, just like Tanya who could not intervene when her mother was hit because she was too small. In the film *Big* Tom Hanks longs to be big. In truth he longs to be tall and an adult, a grown-up. If you as a child longed to be big or bigger or to have substance don't be surprised that you have made that happen. The strongest force in every human is that our body has to act in a way that matches our thinking. When you long and wish for something your body finds a way to express that longing physically and it often does it in an unwanted way because we are so unspecific in our longing. It is never too late to undo and reverse this.

Solution
Repeat the following until you believe them:

- I am significant.
- I am important.
- I matter.
- I have a big heart and intellect and a slim, fit body.
- I am an adult and my body is slender and strong.
- Now that I am a grown-up I am free to stop growing and to feel good about being me.

Angry Eaters

Fiona's parents had a very bitter divorce and fought in front of her. She was traumatised by their rage and began to comfort eat. She gained an enormous amount of weight very quickly. The weight clearly had a role, function and purpose. It was telling her parents that she was deeply unhappy and that something was wrong. When we cannot open our mouths and tell people what is bothering us our body must take on this job. In Fiona's case her weight was saying, 'Look at what you have done to me and look how unhappy you are making me'. One of the keys to having inner peace and emotional wellbeing is to express your hurt as close to it occurring as possible. When I was training to be a therapist we were taught that one of the ways that madness is defined is in the length of time it takes to express a hurt or grievance. Become used to expressing your hurt out loud so that your body does not have to express it in a disguised or abnormal way for you. When you express your feelings you don't need to swallow them with food. Using food to push feelings down doesn't work. When you can't say it out loud because it's your boss or relative who's upset you, lock yourself in the bathroom and run the taps so you can say out loud what you're upset about rather than comfort eating. You *must* express it verbally.

Although Fiona was grown up and had long ago left home she kept the excess weight. Its function and role were still so imbedded in her. Discovering what it was all about freed her.

Solution

If you identify with this client's case history then use the effective statements below, repeatedly, to achieve freedom from the bad habits you have developed:

- I express myself easily so my body doesn't have to do it for me.
- I understand my feelings and deal with them.
- I am free to have a fit, healthy body.
- I express it instead of eating it.
- I am at peace with myself.
- I forgive and let go and am physically and emotionally healthy and well.
- I am letting go of the excess weight and its role, function and purpose simultaneously.
- Chewing gum helps angry eaters. We have receptors in our jaws that respond to chewing by releasing relaxing feelings. Gum gives you the same relaxed feeling as comfort food but without the calories.

Nell was slim when she married her rock star husband. He made it very clear to her that she was expected to look perfect all the time. He was very controlling about what she ate and if she appeared to gain any weight at all he was critical and cold with her. She began to feel that he did not love her, only what she looked like, and within a year she gained a lot of weight. It was her way of saying love me as I am.

I had another client, Susie, who was married to an even more famous actor. She began to live a Hollywood life and hated it. She found it hard to look beautiful every day and told me that she felt she was in a competition with all the other wives to look sensational 24/7. She realised she was in a race to stay slim and pretty and not only could she not win this race, she couldn't even reach the finishing line. It constantly moved beyond her reach as she was surrounded by younger and more beautiful women. She found the pressure so overwhelming that she became a compulsive eater and gained a lot of weight which took her out of the competition completely. Nell and Susie could be classed as emotional eaters but in each case their anger towards their husbands and the situation they were in drove the overeating, and of course the anger is an emotion.

Solution

Use the following statements to enforce the right messages:

- I accept myself as lovable and I am filled and nourished by things other than food.
- I am unique and lovable. I love my body, I treat it with respect.
- I eat in a way that nourishes my body and makes me feel and look great.
- I am unique. I don't need to compete with or compare myself to anyone.
- I matter as a person.

Particularly with habitual and emotional eating, there is also the issue that for many of us food equates to love. I had a wonderful grandmother who absolutely loved me but showed me that love through food. The minute I walked in her door she would get out the cake tin and offer me all kinds of goodies that she had bought or baked just for me. As a child I was delighted by this, as a twenty-year-old trying to control my weight I refused them and she was very hurt and offended. She took my refusal personally. I soon noticed that the instant I entered her door I wanted to eat cakes. If she wasn't home I would help myself from the same tin. Even if I had had a full meal beforehand I still wanted them.

I had built an association with her house and food that was very strong. I had an issue with food for years partly through being loved with food. It is not an exaggeration to say it ran my life and I am so happy that it no longer does.

Identify Your Eating Habits and Take Action

Addictive eaters can be very successfully cured once they have identified the foods that are triggers for them. They can break their addiction by choosing to replace specific foods with something similar but healthy and not chemically addictive. My blog (www.marisapeer.blogspot.com) has some great alternatives to junk food. Many of us have addictive traits, it's hard to eat one chocolate, one peanut or one crisp and many of us find once we start we can't stop. Instead of berating yourself for having an addictive trait you can absolutely use this to your benefit. It is easy to get addicted to good habits going to the gym: exercising, eating fruit, even drinking water. I have many celebrity clients who have what I call 'positive addictions' – they can't miss yoga or a gym session or they go everywhere with a water bottle as they feel 'addicted' to it. I have worked with many ex-addicts who became addicted to extreme sports instead of drink and drugs. You don't need to behave in an extreme way but you can learn very quickly to replace every negative habit or addiction with a new positive one. The next chapter, Ending Cravings, will show you exactly how to do this.

Emotional, angry and **destructive eaters** will find a lasting cure as they deal with their feelings and take charge of their thoughts, beliefs and language. Emotional eaters need to feel nourished by things other than food. Destructive eaters must feel safe as well as slender. Angry eaters need to express their emotions instead of swallowing them. Overeating is a learned response that you are unlearning through this programme. The first chapters of this book have already begun the process of lasting change for emotional, destructive and angry eaters and the next chapter will continue this.

Ignorant and **habitual eaters** are easier to cure because human behaviour often falls into patterns – we are creatures of habit. However we can choose good habits.

Habits are easier to break if you replace them with something new. To break a habit you need to:

1   Be convinced you can do it.
2   Make a decision to start now.
3   Initiate it.
4   Absolutely persist.
5   Allow yourself to feel a sense of accomplishment and achievement.

Your habits, beliefs, actions and thoughts are yours to change. Only you can do it. Physical cravings ruin diets, figures and lives. You can break the vicious circle, it's really not that hard. I did it and I have never looked back, neither have my clients.

Disclaimer – Although the methods and techniques in this book can really help how you feel about yourself and your relationship with food, if you have an extreme eating disorder such as anorexia, bulimia or body dysmorphia, please seek additional help from your doctor or a recognised professional body.

Leave Childhood Eating in Your Childhood

Many of my clients report that they begin each day determined to do well on a new eating plan. They stay on target until late afternoon, and then at around 4 o'clock they lose their resolve and begin to crave cakes, biscuits or sweets. In therapy they very often recall coming home from school to a snack of something sweet or stodgy. Many adults have programmed themselves to recreate this scenario by eating the same foods at the same time of day. We have taste receptors in the mouth that link certain tastes to certain sensations. That is why we always crave foods like toast, ice cream, biscuits, cakes, chocolate, desserts, cereal with milk, etc. Few people crave comfort food in the form of salads, vegetables, sushi or steamed fish. We have no memories of these foods being given to us as a treat or comfort so we can't re-enact anything by eating them. Food is linked to memories, both good and bad, that's why many adults hate semolina, tapioca or Brussels sprouts because of the memories of being made to eat them at school. These memories are still having an effect years later.

Overeating is a search for security: a need to recreate the secure feeling we got as children when we were held and fed and all our needs were met. We felt loved, secure, safe, content and significant and we got attention and time from our mother. By eating foods that are similar in sweetness and texture to the foods we ate as babies, we are trying to reactivate the memory of feeling secure and loved: we are looking to find the feeling in food but it's a search that does not work.

Emotional eaters often want to eat food linked to nice memories to recreate the memory along with the sensation. Emotions are very linked to food and many people who eat sugary fatty foods are searching for the emotional memory the food had for them. Smell is by far the strongest of our five senses and is absolutely linked to memory, followed by taste, hence the smell of freshly baked bread or cake or chocolate will bring back memories, as will the taste of these foods. Equally the smell of boiled cabbage can remind us of being back in the school dining room and the taste of something we were forced to eat like cod liver oil can bring up horrible memories.

When we continuously reward children with food we set up a

pattern in the brain that wires it to believe food makes everything better and is a cure all. We reward children with sweets, snacks and desserts then they learn to associate these foods with feeling better. Food can distract an unhappy child and instantly make things better because children's lives are so simple therefore an ice cream creates instant gratification. Lucy falls over, you buy her an ice cream, she is distracted and happy again. As an adult if Lucy falls out with her boyfriend she buys a big tub of ice cream believing it will still have the same effect, but it can't. As adults our lives are not simple and we cannot find instant gratification in food. It can't make anything better. If you lost your job and your partner and you were describing your feelings of devastation to a friend who replied, 'Here's a chocolate bar, that will make you better', you would find this insensitive and ridiculous. A chocolate bar is not a cure all to an adult. Adults don't need instant gratification, we need the long term gratification of liking our bodies and being healthy.

As an adult you cannot find comfort, distraction, friendship or love in food. If you could, believe me, you would have done so by now.

When children go on long trips it is so easy to distract them with food and it is hard not to do this on a long train, car or plane journey. So many habitual eaters cannot do a long trip without stocking up with sweets and snacks just like when they were children. You can break all of these patterns. Reward yourself with a magazine and an hour to yourself to read it. Buy healthy fruit to snack on.

For many people Christmas and Easter mean lots of chocolate while summer means ice cream because we have programmed ourselves to link a particular food to a particular event. Human behaviour is not random, it is heavily patterned. We set up patterns in our brain, but it is *your* brain and you can change any pattern. By doing the exercises in this book you can break these patterns forever.

If you sabotage your diet at teatime or get those early evening cravings for stodgy, fatty or sugary foods the way to stop them and to stop looking for comfort in food is to say to yourself out loud several times:

- I am not a child. I refuse to eat like one.
- I don't need that. I don't eat that. I don't do that.
- I don't need nursery food.
- Cake cannot make me feel better.
- Food cannot solve any problems.
- I have a healthy adult relationship with food now and always.

Every time you do this you are moving away from a negative learned response and rewiring your brain for success, so do it frequently and enthusiastically.

If you want to have a slender adult body you need to eat like a healthy adult. If you were travelling in first or business class you would enjoy all the luxury grown-up food served in first class. You would not ask the stewardess to go into economy and get you the children's chips, beans and chicken nuggets, because you would feel silly. Imagine being at a glamorous event with two buffet tables, one for the adults laden with lobster, seafood, chicken, Parma ham, exotic salads, fresh mango, papaya and berries. The other is laid out for the children with chips and ketchup, sticky doughnuts with vivid pink icing melting in the heat, bowls of crisps and sweets in psychedelic colours and those bright blue and pink crushed ice drinks. Which would you choose? Imagine how odd it would be to eat all the children's food with all the children while the other adults looked on baffled by your behaviour and choices.

When my daughter was very small and had birthday parties the other children's parents always came along to supervise their toddlers. I would provide grown-up food and wine for the adults and smiley face biscuits, crisps, sweets, egg mayonnaise sandwiches and sausages on sticks for the children. Every now and again an adult would hover over the children's table and eat all their sweets as quickly as possible looking horribly uncomfortable. I have done this myself, before I sorted out my eating habits, and I always hated the feeling afterwards.

It is so much nicer to eat and feel like an adult than to be stuck in that vicious circle of eating to feel better and ultimately feeling worse.

Ending Cravings

So far we have been working on ending habits and cravings that originate in the mind. Tests show that physical addictions are much easier to cure than mental ones. By now you have done a great job of resolving psychological cravings and are ready to get rid of the physical cravings too.

How to End Carbohydrate Cravings

One of the downfalls to any healthy eating plan is a craving for certain foods that are chemically addictive and change our moods. One of the biggest factors in food craving is a lack of serotonin. Serotonin is a very important and essential hormone which elevates mood, which is why it's known as the happy hormone. Research has found that bulimics, compulsive eaters and alcoholics lack the required levels of serotonin. Indeed, alterations in the levels of serotonin can actually trigger eating disorders. Low levels of serotonin are also linked to depression.

Researchers have found that carbohydrates are essential to the production and regulation of serotonin and serotonin is essential to keep our moods regulated. Serotonin has been central to studies investigating the causes and treatment of depression. Several anti-depressant drugs work by artificially increasing levels of serotonin in the brain and are designed to make serotonin stay in the bloodstream for longer, thereby keeping our moods and energy levels higher. They are known as selective serotonin re-uptake inhibitors or SSRIs. Prozac is a well-known SSRI.

Studies have shown that people eating a high carbohydrate diet produce more serotonin and are more relaxed as a result. This is why so many people with eating disorders absolutely crave stodgy carbohydrates in the form of bread, cakes and biscuits. They are not necessarily craving that particular food, they are actually craving the serotonin boost it gives them. Alcoholics who come off alcohol frequently crave carbohydrates and sugar to replace the sugar rush they got from alcohol. They also crave fatty snacks, as foods high in fat also appear to increase serotonin levels.

There are people I call 'carbohydrate cravers' who have to eat a certain amount of stodgy carbohydrates to keep their moods steady and balanced. Carbohydrate cravers experience a change in their mood in late afternoon or early evening and as their mood changes they begin to crave sweet and starchy foods. Protein does not elevate their mood even though serotonin uses ingested protein in its production.

People who eat quickly and cram food into their mouth without really tasting it are actually craving the high they get from serotonin. Just like a drug addict they are looking for the feeling but in food rather than drugs. They are not thinking about what they eat or savouring each bite and enjoying the process, there is no interaction with the food. They are eating to get the feeling of mood elevation, to get high on serotonin. Just like any other addiction you have to give up the source of the addiction, to see it as a poison for your body and keep away from it. Many people self medicate with food without even realising it. They use food to sedate themselves, to tranquillise themselves, to feel better and to elevate their mood. They always use stodgy carbs to do this as they are the only foods that can do this. Starchy carbohydrates including pasta, bread, biscuits, rice and potatoes stimulate sedative-like brain chemicals; they would not get that feeling from copious amounts of berries or fish. A warm milky drink before bed releases sedative brain chemicals as does eating a stodgy meal.

Does this pattern sound familiar? You may recognise yourself here, you certainly don't need to be bulimic or a compulsive eater to have this problem. Many people find they can eat sensibly and retain control all day but come teatime or the evening they have a longing for cakes, bread and sweets and nothing else will do. They are comfort foods. When we feel low we want puddings, toast, sweets, biscuits or other starchy foods. Many people who are unwell also crave starchy foods for the serotonin boost it gives them. Men do this even more than women, when they have flu or a hangover they want to eat what I call nursery food. Women want to overeat on stodgy carbs when they are unhappy, anxious, stressed or feel unloved.

When one of my friends died I was so sad I could hardly eat, but when I did resume eating I only wanted to eat chips. My other friends who were also mourning our loss and who eat a diet similar to mine (yes, I have converted almost all my friends) reported cravings for white bread and cakes. If you react like this you can naturally increase your serotonin levels with healthier foods that encourage your body to make more serotonin. The five best healthy foods that help the body increase its production of serotonin are coriander, bananas, eggs, avocados and turkey. I make sure I have scrambled eggs with coriander for breakfast three or four times a week and I eat a banana every day to keep my serotonin levels up.

Bananas are full of B vitamins and tryptophan which increase dopamine levels. A lack of dopamine is also linked to depression. Serotonin is made from the amino acid tryptophan; certain foods are tryptophan rich, especially turkey and bananas but also eggs, avocados and coriander. You can easily find a way of incorporating those five foods into your diet and if you don't like one of them just have more of the others. Coriander is a delicious herb that you can grow yourself and the other four foods are very inexpensive.

Sunlight also helps the brain make serotonin so make sure you get outside more, especially in winter. Many people crave starchy carbs in the winter and link it to the poor weather. They are correct to a degree as the lack of light in the winter can cause the brain to make less serotonin and the starchy carbs are giving them a serotonin boost. Eating more starchy carbs is never the answer because when you eat junk food and white flour it can cause your levels of serotonin to rise and drop so fast that this can actually trigger eating disorders and food cravings. Chewing food slowly can help maintain serotonin levels and also reduces appetite. Another factor that diminishes serotonin is aspartame, an artificial sweetener that is used particularly in diet drinks and low-fat snack foods as a sugar substitute to keep the calorie content of the product down. Reducing the fat reduces the calories but also makes the flavour bland so sweetners or sugar substitutes are added to increase the flavour. However, when aspartame is combined with carbs it slows down the brain's production of serotonin.

To end carb cravings and naturally increase serotonin

- Eat coriander, bananas, eggs, turkey and avocados regularly.

- Get outside in natural daylight especially in the winter.

- Chew food slowly to trigger serotonin.

- Take vitamin B6 and B complex supplements as it also helps to make serotonin.

- Don't eat junk food, white flour and sugar as they disrupt and alter your serotonin levels.

- Limit and restrict your consumption of aspartame.

If you stop eating refined and processed carbohydrates you will eventually stop craving them. It's the same with all addictions: stop feeding the monster and it will die. Your serotonin levels will balance out and become more stable when you stop the cycle of eating or bingeing on rubbish, and the rush of insulin and glucose it brings, followed by the dramatic drop that sets the vicious craving cycle off again.

Certain carbs can have such a powerful and detrimental effect on our bodies. Several new studies have shown that bulimics who are taken off all wheat products completely can recover from bulimia, but resuming the consumption of wheat can cause a relapse at any time. Bulimics mostly crave sugar and refined carbohydrates. I have worked with hundreds of bulimics but have yet to meet a bulimic who craved grilled fish and broccoli or hard-boiled eggs and tomatoes. They always report the same thing, 'Once I have one bowl of cereal I have five more, the minute I start on bread I eat the whole loaf, as soon as I open the biscuits or crisps I eat them until they are gone.' No one has ever said to me, 'Once I start on a whole chicken I eat it all and then another one and once I start on a punnet of blueberries I eat ten more punnets.' This is because real food satisfies us quickly whereas refined food is so full of chemicals and so altered in the refining process it drives us to crave more and need more which is why it needs to be avoided most of the time.

Another reason to steer away from refined carbs is that research has found that children who eat high carbohydrate breakfast cereals get hungry again before lunch and want to snack on junk food. These children consume more calories overall than children who have a protein breakfast. The children on the protein-based breakfast ate more moderately all day and had much better concentration and attention.

Bread may be delicious, whether it's French, Italian or Arabic, but it is still glue. Glue? Yes, it is flour and water and anyone who's spent time playing with children knows how to make glue from flour and water. I still have books from my childhood with pictures I stuck in with glue my mother made from flour. Forty years later they are still stuck down.

To see what I mean by glue, if you take a piece of bread (about 3 inches) and roll it in your palms you will find that as the moisture comes out of it, it will become solid like Play-Doh. Play-Doh is just what it says it is – dough with lots of toy-coloured dyes, and it lasts in those little pots for ages. This is what it is like in your stomach – hard and useless as a source of nutrition and hard for the body to digest. My grandmother once made Christmas decorations out of dough. Every year she got them out and hung them on the tree, eventually they fell apart but they didn't decompose the way live food like fruit and vegetables would, because modern dough made from processed refined flour is dead, inert, lifeless food. It's dead before you eat it and dead and inert in your body whereas fruit and vegetables are live healthy food.

Another reason women in particular should avoid highly processed carbohydrates and sugary foods is that they can quadruple the risk of birth defects. Pregnant women who eat a lot of breakfast cereals, white bread, white rice or chocolate biscuits put their babies at risk of abnormalities. Tests compared diets of 454 mothers with babies with birth defects against 462 women with healthy babies. The risk of birth defects increased four–fold in women who ate high levels of sugar and highly refined carbohydrates like chocolate biscuits and breakfast cereals, and potatoes. Researchers believe the high level of glucose these foods release, quickly giving a massive sugar rush followed by a low, may overwhelm the baby in the womb interfering with key development stages.

An expert from an important birth defects monitoring programme states, 'There is an association between neural tube defect risk and the glycaemic index of the mothers. The risk doubles in women eating a high carbohydrate diet in pregnancy. In obese pregnant women eating a high carbohydrate diet the risk quadruples.'

Refined carbohydrates are even linked to infertility, not just because all the pesticides and chemicals in refined white flour are so disruptive to your body (as are the trans fats used in baked goods and convenience food) but also because polycystic ovary syndrome, which is a common cause of infertility and irregular and painful periods, is caused by insulin resistance or pre diabetes. You may be able to reverse polycystic ovary syndrome by eliminating refined carbs from your diet. Remember Karen, the little girl in Step Three who suffered from epilepsy and had to choose not to eat foods that made her fits worse? In an experiment at Great Ormond Street Hospital, a group of epileptic children who were having up to eighty seizures a day were put on a high-fat and low-carbohydrate diet. When all bread, cereals, rice, potatoes and snack foods were banned, the diet proved to have dramatic results. Within days the fits were reduced to between two and twelve per day. The results showed that after three months many of the children had a 75 per cent reduction in seizures, 50 per cent were able to reduce medication dramatically. Some came off medication altogether and the children showed a 75 per cent improvement in alertness, awareness and responsiveness. The tests showed that the low-carbohydrate diet changed the metabolism of these children for the better.

These children had baked goods made out of almond flour and all of their parents reported that the effort involved in changing their diet was absolutely worth it as the results were profound. The diet and test results are available from www.gosh.nhs.uk.

No one fully understands why epileptic children cannot metabolise refined carbohydrates but these tests do prove that for some people starchy and refined carbohydrates have a destructive effect on their metabolism. Researchers are beginning to link the rise in violent crime, mental disorders, ADD (Attention Deficit Disorder) and other children's ailments to the West's growing consumption of processed foods and refined carbohydrates.

I have been telling my clients for twenty years to avoid refined flour, and whenever anyone says to me, 'How come you are so slim yet you eat a lot?' I always reply, 'I don't eat flour'. You don't have to give it up completely but you can choose to limit its intake. More and more doctors and dieticians are coming to the same conclusion and I believe that soon the link between refined flour and obesity will be proved. We can already see it works by looking at Thai, Japanese and Chinese people where they have a very low percentage of overweight people. An Asian diet does not include flour, they do not eat bread or pasta and many of the noodles they eat are rice noodles. Yet Thai, Japanese and Chinese people who live in America and eat an American diet do have weight problems. The most overweight Americans are African Americans but Africans are not fat and they don't eat wheat flour only maize. African Americans are the poorest Americans and eat a diet that is often 80 per cent wheat products. To me that is heartbreaking and so unnecessary. Most people who are overweight eat 80 per cent of their daily food intake in the form of refined flour of which 50 per cent is bread alone, the other 30 per cent comes from pasta, cakes, biscuits, crackers, noodles, pastry and snacks. Imagine that, eating 80 per cent of your daily food from a source that was not even put on the planet for you but exists as a food source for cattle. Half of the world eats 50 per cent of its calories every day from bread, and 70 per cent of the food we eat today is food our ancestors never ate.

In our grandparents' day most people ate about thirteen different food types in one day, the variety came from fruits, vegetables, proteins and starches. Today we eat only six to eight different types of food but the majority of these come from one food group; refined carbohydrates and primarily white bread, cakes, biscuits and sugary snacks.

Something to stick in your mind!

To get an idea of what bread is like in your body, take some bread or flour, put it in a big mixing or salad bowl, add some water and mix it all up with your hands until it resembles a paste. Really play with it and feel the texture and consistency, eat a little of it if you can bear to then

---

leave it in the bowl on your kitchen counter for about two weeks and watch what happens to it as this will help put you off wheat.

Every day imagine that sticky mass in your stomach and intestines, imagine what it is doing to your body. Don't wash it off your hands completely and you will notice it sets like concrete. That is just how it is in your body. Have you ever left half-finished cereal bowls until you come back from work in the evening and noticed how the residue of cereal has set like cement? Well, imagine if that's what it was like in your body.

I am a great believer that you don't want to hear this, you need to see it. You will believe it when you see it so take a lump of the paste you have made from water and bread or water and flour and stick some paper together with it then stick another piece of paper to the wall with this glue. It will stay stuck like this for weeks, even years. If you love to have bread and cereal for breakfast leave the paper stuck to you kitchen wall and leave the bowl of glue out on your kitchen worktop to remind you of what you have been eating.

If you always have sandwiches at work because it's easy, remind yourself that it is not at all easy for your body to digest by having a bowl or container of this gluey mess on your desk or in your drawer to look at and remind you of what it really is. Use a lump of it to stick a piece of paper to your wall or filing cabinet to reinforce just how sticky it is. If you can't do this, stick it to a book and keep it in your desk or locker or bag to jog your memory. I always do this at my seminars – make up a bowl of glue and stick some to the wall. At my last seminar one of the participants told me that when her mother was wallpapering she ran out of wallpaper paste so she improvised with flour and water and found it just as effective as, and much cheaper than, buying wallpaper paste. That really is food for thought.

Remembering what that gluey paste looks like, close your eyes and imagine you can see inside your body. Look at your stomach and intestines and imagine that paste coating everything. Look how hard your poor body is working to try to extract some form of nutrition from it and just when it might have made a bit of an inroad you put in some more and this goes on all day. No wonder your body protests with gas, distension heartburn and fatigue. Ask your body how it feels to be filled up with glue and to have to work so hard to try and digest it. When you get a message back from your body (and you will if you do this properly and stick with it for a few minutes) you can make a commitment to stop punishing your body this way and to respect it. So go ahead and memorise this then close your eyes and imagine it now.

How to End Sugar Cravings

If you have sugar cravings it is important to remember that highly refined sugar is not food at all, it is a chemical. Sugar creates an acidic environment in your body which then has to produce more fat cells to keep the acid away from your organs. Sugar makes you fat, rots your teeth, disrupts your digestion and is extremely addictive. Sugar also feeds anxiety and depression and is toxic to the lining of blood vessels, leading to plaque.

When you crave something sweet and sugary you can satisfy the craving with naturally sweet foods that won't have this effect on your body: figs, dates, berries and other fruits, and with creamy soya yogurts and shakes and sugar-free nut, seed and hemp bars. Small grapes can stop a sugar craving and soaked blanched almonds are very sweet too. In addition, almonds and pumpkin seeds are full of B vitamins and zinc, which is a benefit since low levels of zinc are linked to depression which leads to comfort eating. Zinc supplements also help you keep off sugary foods. To increase your zinc levels you can eat more prawns as they are naturally rich in zinc. Another way to keep your sugar levels naturally balanced is to eat cinnamon – half a teaspoon a day of ground cinnamon reduces sugar levels in the blood, and you can add it to oats or soya milk, put it in fruit smoothies or stewed fruit or add it to curries.

Many people who crave sugar are low in magnesium, chromium and manganese, so take a combined calcium, magnesium and chromium supplement to better absorb the magnesium. Magnesium-rich foods will also lessen sugar cravings. These include dates, apples, avocados, Brazil nuts, almonds, celery, parsley and fish. A diet deficient in magnesium, calcium and potassium can cause weight gain as well as sugar cravings.

I am not a fan of salt but eating something salty can often end a carb and sugar craving. Roasted sunflower seeds with tamari sauce, tahini and sauerkraut are good healthy salty tastes. I used to eat masses of sweets and confectionery and would buy them every day. I would never have believed that fruit could replace chocolate and initially when I craved chocolate eating grapes was not the same. However, I made a decision to give up sugar and using the same methods I am teaching you I gave it up very easily for three months. I decided to eat it again on my birthday and was amazed to find that I didn't like it in the same way I used to, it was no longer that enjoyable and I have never craved it since. I only wish I had done it years earlier.

Another factor to consider as a reason to give up refined sugar is that it seriously ages your skin. Sugar molecules attach themselves to collagen causing the fibres to become rigid, stiff and inflexible. This in turn increases wrinkles, particularly frown lines, laughter lines and nose-to-mouth lines, and makes them deeper and more pronounced. So sugar will make your face prematurely lined, saggy and jowly whereas a diet low in refined sugar will leave you with a more youthful and firm complexion.

How to End Crisp Cravings

We delude ourselves that crisps are healthy potatoes cooked in sunflower oil and a reasonable snack. The truth is most crisps are made up of trans fat and masses of chemicals. Many crisps are not made of real potatoes at all but of a reconstructed mashed potato mix and a cocktail of additives, there is nothing natural about them.

Fat burning!

If you want to put yourself off crisps for life take some regular potato crisps, get some matches and, holding a crisp over a metal tray, light one crisp at a time and watch how slowly it burns and how much fat drips off it. When the crisp is half burned place it on the tray until it burns out and watch the fat drip off, you can get a full teaspoon of fat from just one crisp. You would be unable to eat that fat from the teaspoon but you are eating it every time you eat crisps and your body has to deal with all that fat. The reason crisps burn so slowly is because they are pure fat and it takes that fat some time to burn. It would be incredibly difficult to set fire to a potato but you can light a crisp and watch it burn. It will go black and the smoke that comes off it is horrible because of all the fat and chemicals. Really focus on the smell, the fat dripping off the crisps and the smoke and you will feel different about crisps forever.

I was teaching this to some children and one little boy wrote to me to say he has never eaten crisps since. Obviously you must do this with your children – don't let them do this alone and make sure you have a bowl of water to hand.

Next take a Pringle and place it in your mouth on your tongue, don't bite into it just leave it there and you will feel all the fat and chemicals starting to saturate your mouth. If you leave it for a while it will literally stick to the roof of you mouth. Try it, it's horrible and will change your concept of what crisps are, you will never look at them the same way again. Instead of crisps you can snack on olives, Japanese soy beans, seeds, fruit, nut and seed bars, vegetables with dips or hummus, unsalted nuts and natural popcorn.

You can see a video of a crisp burning on my website www.marisapeer.com

How to End Cravings For Bad Fats and Junk Food

Don't even think about replacing dairy products with margarine. Margarine is but ONE MOLECULE away from being PLASTIC. To prove this to yourself, buy a tub of margarine and leave it in your garage or a shaded area outside. Within a couple of days you will notice that no flies, rodents or insects will go near it (that should tell you something) and it doesn't rot or smell because it has no nutritional value; nothing will grow on it. Even micro organisms won't grow on trans fats. They don't decompose – why?

Because it is nearly plastic, it's what I call chemical, fake food or non-food. It's about as real and healthy as the tub it came in and you wouldn't melt and eat that, would you? Would you eat a food that rats and flies won't touch? Of course not, so keep that in mind and it will help you to say no to it. It's a good idea to let your children monitor the tub of plastic margarine in the garden as it will help them stop eating it too. You don't need to feel any sense of shame about eating margarine prior to today, because you didn't have this information before now. Food companies don't exactly want you to know how unnatural and scarily unhealthy some of their foods are. I get so cross when diet experts try to shame people about their weight and make them feel humiliated about how they have been eating. You didn't manufacture this non-food, spend a fortune advertising it and then place it in the shops and pretend it's healthy, slimming and full of vitamins. You bought it because you got conned and brainwashed by the adverts just as they wanted you to be, and if anyone should feel a sense of shame it's the companies that produce and market this stuff. Don't beat yourself up – just stop buying it, and remember it isn't just margarine, many other foods contain trans fats including fast food, junk food, snack food, biscuits, pies, pastries, cakes, crackers, chips, crisps, powdered hot drinks and ready meals.

Remind yourself that it's almost plastic and if it's unfit for rats and flies it has to be unfit for you and your family. Rats know that and now you know it too. It doesn't stop you gaining weight, either; trans fats are linked to weight gain, cancer, diabetes and heart disease. So look at that untouched plastic in your garden and remind yourself it's a chemical not a food and it can make you ill and fat. It belongs in the bin, not in your body. Your body cannot break down and digest plastic (instead it wraps it in fat and stores it in your body), so eating so-called slimming spreads and diet foods can make you fatter even if the calories are low. If you don't have a garden or balcony you can put it by your front door or on a windowsill. Don't worry, it won't attract insects it will repel them and now you can be just as repelled. You can eat Pure, which is an organic soy spread, or organic olive-oil spread stocked by most supermarkets and health food shops. Don't eat foor that is made in a refinery.

Milk Sucks – How to End Dairy Cravings

Just as we have been brainwashed into eating cereals, which are essentially cattle feed, and believing they are a healthy food, we have also been brainwashed into believing that dairy produce is a healthy food for humans. I am opposed to any diet that promotes eating a lot of dairy food. Milk contains insulin growth factor (IGF) a growth hormone, and oestrogen and progesterone, so consuming any dairy product will have an effect on your body's natural hormone levels. Cow's milk is not a food for humans at all, it is a product packed full of growth hormones that promote cell division and it is designed to nourish calves through their biggest growth spurt and to give them a 300 per cent weight gain within a year. A calf's body weight doubles in six weeks then triples until within two years a 90 pound calf weighs 2000 pounds, while a human baby triples its birth weight in about twelve months. A calf is almost the same size as its parent in less than a year, while it takes human children about sixteen years to become the same size as their parents. Any food that can encourage a 300 per cent weight gain is to be avoided like the plague by humans. It cannot be a coincidence that countries that do not consume dairy have the leanest people and countries where the most dairy is consumed have the fattest people, because milk is designed to make you grow. The chemical and hormonal structure of milk stimulates huge growth in calves, it literally sends a message to their cells that says GROW! When adult humans drink cow's milk it sends a similar message to their already fully grown bodies: GROW! I have worked with many very overweight clients who have had dramatic and permanent success in dropping a lot of weight just by eliminating dairy produce.

A mother's milk delivers antibodies to her baby. Cow's milk delivers the cow's antibodies, hormones and chemicals to humans. You can buy low-fat and even non-fat cow's milk but you cannot buy non-growth hormone milk because milk literally is a growth hormone that promotes cell division and rapid growth. It makes many humans grow bigger than they were ever meant to be because it was not designed for humans. None of us wants to grow and develop like a cow. Dairy produce is the cause of allergies in many people and has been linked to the occurrence of headaches, sinusitis, indigestion, nausea, diarrhoea, cramps, irritable bowel syndrome, ear infections and breathing problems. The oestrogen and progesterone in milk can be a cause of acne, eczema and many other skin conditions. When you consume dairy produce you are consuming a hormonal delivery system.

Dairy foods can be disruptive to humans when consumed excessively and have been linked to infertility, prostate cancer and breast tumours. Some researchers believe that the insulin growth factor in milk and lactose, the type of sugar found in milk, can over stimulate the production of hormones which may encourage tumour growth. The higher our levels of insulin growth factor, the higher risk we have of developing certain cancers. In some Scandinavian countries women who have had breast tumours are advised to have a dairy-free diet permanently. In China they call breast cancer rich white women's illness. The Chinese who have breast cancer are mostly those who eat a Western diet. In Asian countries, where they eat very little dairy, breast cancer rates are the lowest in the world. Apparently, Japanese people can smell undigested milk in the guts of Westerners, and you may remember me mentioning that singers routinely avoid milk as it is so mucus forming it has a negative effect on their voice.

Non-organic milk is polluted with hormones, pesticides, steroids, antibiotics and is full of synthetic hormones. In modern intensive factory-farming cows are kept in milk all year round by being injected with bovine growth hormones. A cow should produce 10lb of milk daily but the hormones they are injected with make them produce up to a 100lb of milk daily. In factory farming, the cows are milked by machine and the machines extract cow's pus and blood along with the milk. All milk can be 50 per cent mucus and has to be pasteurised to kill the bacteria, but the pasteurising process also kills any beneficial enzymes. Even pregnant cows are milked and this is very unhealthy as that milk is loaded with bovine hormones. Up to two thirds of our milk comes from pregnant cows. It contains thirty-five different hormones and eleven different growth factors. Drinking milk is taking in cows' hormones, synthetic hormones and bovine antibiotics. I avoid cheese and ice cream as they are nothing more than concentrated cows' milk. I used to like ice cream but by seeing it for what it really is it is makes it easier to refuse. If you want to learn more about the negative effects of milk visit www.notmilk.com, www.dumpdairy.com or read *Your Life in Your Hands* by Dr Jane Plant (Virgin Books).

I was on a flight and when the stewardess brought over my meal tray I told her I had ordered a dairy-free meal. The woman next to me said, 'Don't you eat dairy?' 'No,' was my reply. 'But it comes from a cow,' she said. 'Yes, and gorilla milk comes from a gorilla, and dog's milk from a dog and you know what I don't eat that either,' I replied. We have been so brainwashed to believe that milk is good for us but no other animal on the planet drinks the milk of another species. No adult animal on the planet drinks its mother's milk at all. We share 96 per cent of our DNA with chimpanzees but we would never drink ape's milk, yet we drink the milk of a species so vastly different to us and expect our body to digest it.

After the Second World War the Milk Marketing Board heavily promoted milk as a health food and the promotion worked. It is not a health food, it is very unhealthy. Cheese protein has opiates in it and is highly addictive and extremely unhealthy. It is not true that we need extra dairy produce for the calcium needed for healthy bones. A recent study in the May 2005 issue of the journal *Paediatrics* concludes that there is little evidence that increasing dairy produce is the right way to promote bone health in children. Drinking a lot of milk is not the best way to get calcium. Nutrition researchers from Harvard and Cornell Universities in the United States believe that exercise, hormone levels, smoking, hereditary factors, protein intake and most importantly our intake of vitamins D and K matter more than our intake of cow's milk when it comes to osteoporosis and healthy bones. We all need calcium but we don't need excessive amounts of dairy produce in order to get it.

In a study known as 'The China Study', also available as a book,

Dr T. Colin Campbell found that Asians who consume far less dairy than Westerners have one fifth of the bone fractures we have. Asians get their calcium from green leafy vegetables. The countries that consume the most cows' milk have the highest fracture rates and the worst bone health. In Africa, the Masaii are the only tribe among the forty tribes in Kenya and Tanzania who suffer with osteoporosis. The Masaii are also the only tribe who own cattle and drink a lot of milk.

We can actually take in too much dairy. Animal protein, and in particular the protein in milk, makes our blood and tissue more acidic, and in order to neutralise this acid the body pulls calcium from our bones. The most important factors for healthy bones are exercise, especially weight-bearing exercise, and Vitamin D which our bodies get from sunlight. Fifteen minutes of sun exposure on our face and arms will give us enough vitamin D. If you avoid the sun or use sun block you need to take vitamin D supplements unless you regularly eat eggs and oily fish (natural sources of vitamin D).

Children up to the age of ten produce lactase in their bodies naturally, which does break down the lactose (the milk sugar) in milk. After ten it becomes harder for our bodies to process milk, so while small children can tolerate milk adults can't. Therefore you don't need to take milk away from children but adults do not need it and cannot digest it properly. No human can break down the casein, the protein in milk, and many humans (studies say up to 75 per cent) are lactose intolerant, the undigested lactose encourages bacteria growth in our intestines.

When you eat a food that your body can't digest easily it can't absorb much nutrition from it. As a consequence you will still be hungry after eating or hungry again very soon after eating because your body is consuming empty calories and not enough nutrients. If you are still hungry after eating or always hungry it's a sign you are eating food your body cannot work with or efficiently adapt to. Limiting wheat and dairy is not the same as going on a diet. You don't have to go hungry or count calories. You can eat very well and eat very healthy food while shedding weight – you simply have to make other choices.

The worst food combines the two most indigestible foods – wheat and dairy – or more literally glue and mucus: food like pizza, pasta with cheese sauce, cereal with milk, bread and butter, crackers and cheese, milk and cookies, cheese sandwiches, quiche, muffin and cappuccino, toast and hot chocolate. I hate going to coffee houses because they are full of wheat and dairy – cakes, sandwiches, milky drinks and high-sugar drinks – and have few alternatives. Luckily when you cut down on one you naturally cut down on the other.

You do not have to cut milk out of your diet completely but you need to restrict your intake of it. It takes 10 pounds of milk to make just 1 pound of cheese and 12 pounds of milk to make 1 pound of ice cream, so just cutting out cheese will naturally cut a lot of milk from your diet. If you switch to soya yogurt and cream or use olive oil in place of butter and use milk alternatives in place of some regular milk you are already making a huge improvement. If you cannot even conceive of giving up your tea with milk at least buy organic lactose-reduced milk, it is kinder to your digestion but you still need to use it sparingly. Lactose (milk sugar) is also used as a sweetener in many convenience foods, pre-packaged meat and baked goods, it's even in ham so you may be consuming far more of it than you are aware of.

I couldn't get used to black tea so I switched to mint tea, then I found that rice milk tastes great in tea and even my builders drank it and could hardly tell the difference. I used to love milky tea and experimented for some time with milk alternatives. I found that vanilla or plain rice milk is lovely in tea and coffee. Soya milk is a little too nutty but I love soya on oats and I love warm soya milk with cinnamon in it. There are many good milk alternatives; organic soya milk, rice milk, almond milk, oat milk, even milk made from peas and sunflower oil. There are good yogurt alternatives too so cutting down on dairy really isn't as limiting as you'd think. Just make sure you choose the unsweetened varieties.

By the way, eggs are not dairy – cows *do not* lay eggs. Chickens have nothing in common with cows and it amazes me that when

I tell people to restrict dairy they tend to ask if that includes eggs. Again, it is brainwashing. Because shops place eggs next to milk and because the food pyramid puts eggs and milk together we have linked them in our minds. See how easy it is to get brainwashed? But it is also easy to undo it.

So now I've told you about all the negative effects of glue and mucus, I want to show you how strongly your body reacts to foods that contain them. You don't have to eat anything to see the effects, just try the exercises below and they'll give you an astounding illustration of what your body's been trying to tell you for years.

Exercise 1

You can use this technique to establish if you are intolerant to a type of food and to establish which foods don't work for your body.

1   Make a fist and, holding your arm out in front of you, make your arm strong and rigid.

2   Get a friend to push down on the rigid arm to test your strength, while you use all your strength to resist them.

3   Now hold some cheese or milk in your other hand, still making a fist and holding your other arm out in front of you, again make your arm as strong and rigid as you can and have a friend push down on the rigid arm to test your strength, while you use all your strength to resist them. I did this on *Celebrity Fit Club* and the celebrities were astonished at how they lost all their strength when holding cheese, milk shakes or junk food. Even the crew and camera men tried it and the strongest men lost their strength when holding dairy produce, refined carbohydrates and sugar.

---

4 Now reverse the process by holding some natural foods like vegetables or fresh fruit in one hand while making a fist and having someone push down on your other arm. You will stay strong when you hold healthy food in your hand.

When you hold bad food your body sees it as such a threat that you lose all your strength. If your body is depleted just at the idea of these foods then imagine what actually eating them is doing to you. When you hold indigestible foods your body can smell them even if the smell is not at all obvious (remember smell is our most developed sense). Your nose is over your mouth for a reason, we are supposed to smell food before we eat it as all animals do, since the smell of it tells our body if it is digestible.

Also, when you hold, say, cheese in your hand, you are already reacting to it, because you are absorbing its compounds through your skin.

5 You can make this test even more powerful by holding a type of food both good and bad under your nose and smelling it as your friend pushes on your other arm.

Any weakness is telling you that food is indigestible for your body while strength tells you it is a good food for you. Repeat this test over and over again until you get it – that there are some foods that just aren't right for you. Once you have established what they are and have proof of how wrong they are for your body, it will help you to establish and maintain different eating habits and a different body for life.

Exercise 2

Tie a string around your waist and then eat some milk or cheese and monitor what happens. Notice how tight the string gets and how quickly according to the food you are eating. If your stomach is distending too much the food is not breaking down properly in your gut, it is fermenting and putrefying and is the wrong food for you.

Brainwashing For Your Benefit – Since It Works, Make It Work For You Not Against You

As you become more skilled at visualising yourself thinner you can also use your powers of visualisation to turn yourself off bad, unhealthy food. If you want to stop eating and to stop wanting any type of food 'rebrand' it; make the picture wrong, make the descriptive words unpleasant and you will have successfully used your mind to want to eat only the right foods while feeling indifferent to or disgusted by the wrong foods.

We are brainwashed into eating the wrong things by food manufacturers because it's so easy to do and it works. Food manufacturers constantly manipulate us into eating rubbish by giving it healthy and natural-sounding names and it's very effective. I call it re-labelling (although lying is just as good a description for what they do) – using a familiar name to make some unacceptable unhealthy food sound desirable and wholesome: we are encouraged to eat cakes for breakfast because they are called muffins; a sunburst muffin sounds so healthy and kind of sunny, but in truth it is made of flour, sugar, fat, chemicals, preservatives and dried fruit just like cakes. Blueberry muffins are nothing more than blueberry cakes. Breakfast bars are no different to chocolate bars in terms of their nutritional value, and most people would not have a bar of chocolate or a cake for breakfast, yet the sugar and fat in most breakfast cereal bars are the same as in a chocolate bar. We are conned by the branding that says this product is a healthy bowl of cereal in bar. Umm no, actually it really isn't, and who wants a bowl of toxin-, pesticide-, sugar-laden cereal anyway? Many brands of breakfast cereal are nothing more than confectionery. Eating a bowl of cereal is the same as eating a packet of biscuits broken up and drenched in milk. Though Sunny Delight has reinvented itself now, you may remember the original product which sounded like a delightful healthy drink – er, that's odd because it was, in fact, loaded with oil, colours, chemicals and preservatives and had little relation to juice. It was because of this that some supermarkets refused to sell it. Of course if it was called Chemical Delight no one would have bought it as it sounds wrong and conjures up the wrong picture. Likewise fruit juice drinks are full of sugar and colour with little or no fruit in them, and similarly fruit bars tend to be 50 per cent sugar and are not a good alternative to fruit. Crab sticks often have no crab in them at all!

My daughter recently brought home a packet of biscuits that were labelled 'sun-drenched apricot and raisin bars full of goodness' so I read the ingredients and they turned out to be full of sugar, refined syrup, colouring, salt, milk fat, lactose, emulsifiers, preservatives, flour, oh and, of course, some apricots and raisins. Not so full of goodness then. If you want to eat them you can – I didn't stop my daughter eating the bars – but don't kid yourself it's healthy. I picked up a box of cereal bars in a supermarket and they were labelled 'naturally healthy made from the finest Swiss ingredients'. I then read the list of these 'Swiss' 'nutritious' ingredients and the highest one was cane sugar. Since when did sugar cane grow in Switzerland?! It's just more brainwashing and we are totally conned by these companies because they have found a technique that works. The techniques in this book also work but they work in your favour and for your benefit.

Food manufacturers on the whole don't care about your health, they care about making a profit and will use any misleading description to help them sell their products. They can call their foods fresh, pure, natural and wholesome, even if they are none of these things. The labelling is meaningless; it's the list of ingredients that tells the real story. Frequently, the worse the food is the more often it has names with healthy-sounding words incorporating vibrant images such as the sun or 'Swiss' and descriptions like farm enriched, barn fresh, wholesome, fibre-full, etc., and pictures on the packaging to reinforce how healthy they want us to believe it is. Instead of being suckered in by this brainwashing you can use your brilliant brain to defy it, to see that food for the garbage it really is.

When you re-name or rebrand a particular food in your own mind it will lose its desirability and appeal for you. An example of how I do this is calling cola 'osteoporosis in a can', or 'liquid osteoporosis', because carbonated drinks leach calcium from the bones so I am reinforcing the fact that cola has no appeal for me even though I used to love it. An attendee at one of my seminars said that she kept hearing that description in her head and stopped drinking cola overnight when previously she had drunk several cans a day. When my daughter was under four I was amazed at how many of her little friends drank cola. I didn't want to tell her she couldn't have it so instead I put one of her baby teeth in a glass of cola along with a chicken wishbone and a penny coin. Every day she watched with interest and within a week the chicken bone and her tooth had disintegrated and the penny was shining as the acid in the cola had stripped away all the dirt from it. She has always remembered that the acid in cola ruins teeth and bones and she will not drink it, it's no effort for her as she has a mind that is set against it.

You can set your mind against any food if you choose to. Just think about why most people can eat cow but not horse – they just can't imagine eating horse flesh as the picture is all wrong. Many people, including me, can't eat rabbit, snails or pigeon for the same reason. To me snails are so slimy and pigeons are flying vermin, way too disgusting to eat, whereas rabbits are just too cute to eat. I know that sounds illogical but that is how we eat: if the picture in our head looks right we eat it and if the picture looks wrong we don't eat it, it really is as simple as that. I can eat pork but I can't eat suckling pig because the picture it makes in my head is of a cute piglet still suckling from its mother. I can't eat it because I feel like I would be eating a baby, and I don't eat veal for the same reason. Vegetarians don't see a steak or a chop as food, they see a dead animal and can't bring themselves to eat it. You can use this same technique, this same effectiveness to change your whole attitude to food. Think about some of the things you won't eat and think about the reasons why you avoid certain foods. As you do this you will have to conclude it's because you don't like the picture they make in your mind. Very quickly you can feel the same way about foods you were previously unable to resist.

When you stop eating certain foods and see them for what they truly are – fat, pure sugar, or a cocktail of chemicals – they will eventually cease to represent food to you. Call bread 'glue', call milk 'mucus', call cereals 'toxins'. One of the reasons I refer to bread as glue and cattle feed in this book is because this is how I have lost my desire for it. I have done this for so long that now if I go past a bakery I don't see rows of bread, cakes, pastries and biscuits anymore I see baked glue. Dairy produce causes mucus. I tell all my clients that it is full of pus, hormones and growth hormones because imagining cheese as a lump of concentrated mucus and pus works for most people. One of my clients told me he could never drink lattes again after seeing me and he was very happy about that. Do you want some pus on toast? How about some frozen pus in a cornet or some creamy pus in your coffee? No, me neither. Thinking about milk as pus has turned me against it. If you think I am exaggerating, here's the proof: in the EU milk is allowed to be sold when it contains 400,000 somatic pus cells per millilitre. A teaspoon of milk can contain two million pus cells. A cup of milk can contain more than fifty million pus cells. In America the United States Department of Agriculture does not allow milk containing 750 million or more pus cells per litre to cross state lines (how reassuring is that!). When you see a cheese roll as a lump of bleached cattle feed and pesticide containing a filling of concentrated cows' growth hormones its appeal diminishes very quickly. Do this with any kind of food you don't want to crave anymore and you will be free of it. I wouldn't want to eat a doughnut as I now see it as just sugar and batter so it has zero appeal. I don't do this because I am some virtuous zealot, I do it because it's easy and it works. If I wanted biscuits I would eat them but I find it so easy not to and since I ate them by the packet for twenty years I'm glad to be free of them.

When you change your attitude to some foods they no longer mean anything to you and avoiding them is easy. If you cannot eat steak tartare because in your mind the picture you make is raw meat or if you can't eat a raw egg then you already know exactly what I mean. It is easy to learn to do this, to teach yourself to have a different attitude to foods that are best avoided. I used to love pizza, cheese on toast and cheese pasta and now I refuse them without a second thought. It's not a hardship, I don't even like that stuff anymore and I can hardly remember that I used to crave it. I used to mainline jelly babies until I realised they were nothing more than boiled up animal bones with lots of sugar and colorants added. Calling them boiled animal bones ended my desire for them.

I used to buy freshly squeezed orange juice for my daughter until I noticed it said on the bottle in tiny letters 'lightly pasteurised'. Pasteurised means heated to at least 71.7°C and you either heat the juice or you don't, you can't lightly heat it to 71.7. No manufacturer is going to put the words 'lightly heated' on freshly squeezed OJ because it makes the picture in our head all wrong, we all know that heating it up it kills the vitamins and so the point of paying more for freshly squeezed juice is redundant. Once I had pictured it pasteurised I could not picture it as fresh and I don't buy it anymore. I even asked the company why they heated it and they said, 'We do that to kill any bacteria'. When I asked them, 'But doesn't that kill all the vitamins too and anyway you don't boil oranges before sale do you?' they became very vague. Paying £4 a bottle for something that has been rendered as fresh as marmalade is a con.

I want you to think of some foods you would like to stop eating and then change the description of them. Make the words and pictures unattractive and unappealing. For instance, if Swiss chocolate was labelled Third World chocolate its appeal would instantly diminish. Look at the relabelling in the table below for some ideas and apply similar descriptions to the food you are always drawn to and have had trouble resisting.

Breakfast muffin	Nutritionally worthless cake full of sugar fat and preservatives
Breakfast bar	Sugar, flour, chemicals and fat bound up with more fat
Fruit roll up	Sugar, fat and colours rolled together without any fruit
Fruit juice drink	Sugar drink full of colorants and chemicals
Fizzy drink	Liquid osteoporosis/osteoporosis in a bottle/can
Pork scratchings	Solidified fat and chemicals lacking any pork
Fruit chews	Boiled animal bones with added sugar and colours
Potato crisps	Mashed potato mix, chemicals and fat deep fried in more fat
Milk shake	Cows' hormones mixed with colour, chemicals and sugar
Cheese pizza	Glue topped with concentrated cows' mucus and pus
Margarine, slimming spreads and all foods containing trans fats	Plastic non-food, unfit for rats, flies and YOU

How to Eat

I try to make this as easy as possible, knowing that diets fail due to the complication factor. In a nutshell, our bodies are designed to eat everything that was on the planet when we evolved. Nature is very clever and when humans emerged, everything we were meant to eat and everything we could eat was already on the planet in the form of foods that grew or roamed. Our digestive system is designed to digest foods growing on the trees and bushes such as fruits, berries, seeds and nuts and what we could find in the ground such as root vegetables. Any animal that could be caught and its by-products such as its eggs are all digestible. Early man had goats' milk but not cows' milk, which is very indigestible and unhealthy for adults, since goats were much easier to keep than cows and they required a lot less water and pasture. This was the natural food, in fact the *only* food of our ancestors. Their diet was based on fruits, vegetables, nuts and seeds, and though they also ate animal products and animal by-products, they had limited choice and variety depending on what they could catch.

It took humans thousands of years to take the grasses that cattle and wild animals grazed on and make them suitable for human consumption by grinding, milling then baking them. The *Journal of Nutritional and Environmental Medicine* states that the introduction of grains and milk has dramatically changed the way we eat as they are hard to digest. Wheat is not the healthy food we believe it to be, it was imported here from America while potatoes were imported from South America. We have been misled into thinking these foods are healthy when in fact for many people they are unhealthy. Cereals, milk, refined fats and sugar only became staple foods when agriculture was developed. Wheat, a type of grain, is comparatively new to our diets; we started cultivating grains about 10,000 years ago which is new considering man existed without them for well over two million years. Genetically we are almost the same as we were prior to the introduction of grains, and the foods we are best adapted to are the foods freely available to us on the planet at the time we evolved, the food mother nature provided for us: some animal protein, nuts, seeds, fruits, vegetables.

The way to remember how to eat is what I call the 3 Rs

- **Only eat food that grows or Roams.**
- **Only eat food that you could eat Raw.**
- **Only eat food that you Recognise as a natural food.**

Growing and roaming food does not include flour or cereals. Primitive man could not pick wheat and chew it; he/she only ate food that could be eaten raw or cooked speared over an open fire, so cereals were naturally excluded since people 10,000 years ago did not have ovens or mills. Cereals and potatoes are actually toxic in their raw state and dangerous to eat uncooked with the exception of oats, which can be eaten unprocessed and uncooked. You may not want to eat raw eggs or raw meat because they do not seem very palatable, but if you were stranded somewhere and that was the only food available you could eat them and your body would digest them.

Recognisable food means that when you are walking down the aisles of a supermarket you can recognise what the item is made from, for example tuna fish whether fresh, frozen or canned is instantly recognisable. You can recognise eggs, pears, peas, chicken and raw nuts. When you get to bagels, pretzels, cakes, biscuits and packets of Twiglets, cheesy curls, chocolate and jelly beans you can't tell just from looking at them what the raw ingredients are.

When I work with overweight children we do what I call 'warrior shopping', we go down the aisles and imagine what warriors ate and pick similar food and avoid the rest, we only buy recognisable food. Recognisable food does not look very different from its natural state, for instance go for chicken but not chicken roll which is full of cereal and lactose fillers, and buy cut ham rather than ham loaf or processed sliced ham or an even more processed form such as bologna. Eat fillets of fish and shellfish but not fish sticks or ocean sticks or shrimpies, which are full of garbage and bound together with milk protein, fat and sugar. Eat raw unsalted nuts but not tacos, crisps or potato chips as they are full of sugar and bad fats. Eat fresh fruit but not fruit roll ups since they are so full of sugar that they are actually as unhealthy as chocolate bars. Frozen yogurt might sound healthier than ice cream because it's lower in fat, but it is still milk, fat and sugar. Yogurt covered raisins are just fat and sugar-covered raisins.

Food in its most natural state is digestible. Food that grows and roams and does not look too different once it has been prepared and placed on your plate is digestible and in harmony with your body. If you can still recognise it as food you can eat it. Processed cheese doesn't look like food. Cheesy puffs, potato twirls and cheese curls are nothing like food, neither are crisps, sweets and doughnuts. A good rule of thumb is that the more ingredients there are listed on a label the worse the food is and the more indigestible it is. Look for simple ingredients and only about five listings in the ingredients. Natural foods have short ingredient lists; processed foods have long ingredient lists and many chemical names.

Wheat and other cereals in their most basic form are cattle feed – they exist on this planet to feed cattle. The Cereal Board has a lot to answer for in convincing humans to eat cattle fodder, persuading us to eat as if we were cows or sheep. Cereals are promoted and heavily advertised entirely because of the high profit margins involved: cereals are the cheapest food in the world. We have been misled by marketing men into thinking it's a health food. In truth the low-fat, high-carbohydrate diet makes people fat because refining removes the fibre and all the good nutrients from rice, wheat and other cereals. What we are left with is empty calories that promote overeating instead of fullness.

Although unrefined cereals are okay, for example unrefined oats are very healthy, most cereals are loaded with preservatives, pesticides and chemicals. Studies have shown that many stored cereals are contaminated with mycotoxins. How else could you keep them in your food cupboard for months where they don't go mouldy or stale? Even bread has such a long shelf life nowadays that it doesn't go mouldy for weeks. Eating all those chemicals punishes your body. If you want to be slim and healthy disregard forever the food pyramid. Avoid refined foods and white foods such as white rice, white bread or white flour and limit your intake of unrefined cereals. Almost all the overweight people I have worked with have a problem with cereals, after all they are not designed for human consumption. It is only a hundred years since foods became refined and we started to eat foods that dramatically raise our blood sugar levels leaving us hungrier and craving more of the same thing within hours of eating.

The rise in overweight Westerners is linked to the rise in our consumption of bad carbohydrates. The gluten in wheat and other cereals is a big problem as it's hard to digest and can cause allergies, fatigue, bloating, weight gain and Coeliac disease. Modern wheat is modified to contain even more gluten and so genetically tampered with it is indigestible for many people. Digestive problems occur when we are overloaded with wheat by having cereal for breakfast, sandwiches for lunch, pasta for dinner and crackers and biscuits as snacks. There is also a lot of hidden wheat in foods like sausages, burgers, mustard and many sauces. When you eat this way you are consuming a diet of glue all day long. Glue for breakfast, glue for lunch and more glue for dinner and snacks. The word glutinous means sticky and is an adjective derived from gluten. Could you fill up a bowl with flour, oil, pesticides and preservatives, mix it up until it looked like wallpaper paste, like raw pizza dough, and then eat it? No, of course not but that is what you are eating. It may be baked, fried, covered in sauce. It may taste and smell delicious but it is still glue. When your baguette or pizza is broken down in your body it goes back to glue and coats your intestines with a sticky residue so that hours later if you eat some fresh berries or vegetables they will stick to this glue-like matter, this pap coating your gut, and ferment instead of being digested. As a consequence your body is crying out for nutrients not calories. You are full of food but still hungry because your body cannot get enough nutrition from the indigestible food you have put in it.

When we eat digestible food we feel full more quickly and for much longer than when we eat glue. Cows have four stomachs to break down wheat – they need a different digestive tract to deal with wheat. Humans, by comparison, have a much shorter digestive tract and a small stomach. You and I don't have four stomachs but if you eat a wheat-based diet you will begin to look as if you do by the end of each day as your stomach will be bloated and distended. When I ate a lot of bread and cheese my stomach was always very round by the end of each day. It was only flat when I woke up in the morning before eating. It's sad but true that if you eat like a cow you may end up looking like one with a body that has a very big stomach and full of gas with little energy from eating cereal-based products all day. I noticed that my most overweight clients had very large trunks but often normal-sized arms and legs. (Fat stored around the middle is linked to eating too many bad carbohydrates). These patients told me they grazed on food all day and were constantly hungry and lacked energy for any sustainable period of time. They often reported that they had an unnatural amount of gas.

Cows give off more gas that any other animal on the planet. New Zealand actually has a 'fart tax' based on the emissions from each cow on each farm because these emissions are methane which is a greenhouse gas and affects the ozone layer. I am not pointing this out to offend you – I had many of the above symptoms for years so I can identify with it – but because I do believe that if you see cereal as cattle feed it will help you to choose not to eat it very often. One of my clients wrote to me to say, 'I hated you when I left your office but I did remember what you said about not eating like a cow. It stuck in my mind. I have shed four stone and dropped four dress sizes. Guess what I don't hate you anymore. Thank you for making me see sense.'

Think about it – cows, horses and sheep are predominantly all stomach. They graze constantly whereas cats only eat once a day. A lion will kill its prey, which is pure protein, and will leave it when he has eaten enough and he won't eat again for many hours or kill again until he's hungry, even if he is around other prey. Cats will not eat carbohydrates – they are far too smart. They know their bodies cannot digest it so they go hungry instead, because to them going hungry is no worse than actually eating carbohydrates. We need to be as smart and selective about what we eat and focus on the following: cattle eat carbohydrates, cats eat protein. Would you rather be like a cat or a cow? Are you feline or bovine?

Felines are sleek, smart, graceful, lean and fast. Bovines are large, cumbersome and slow. We are like big cats not cows. We have the teeth of carnivores and herbivores because our carnivores teeth are for biting through meat while our herbivore teeth are for chewing vegetables, fruits and nuts. They are not for chewing cud. Have you ever noticed how long cows spend chewing? In addition, cows make between 100 and 150 litres of saliva a day to help break down wheat, whereas humans make about six cups of saliva a day. You need to eat like a celebrity not like a cow. The celebrities I work with avoid wheat and flour as it makes them tired, bloated and gassy.

An Asian diet is more akin to the diet we were meant to eat: they eat rice but no wheat or potatoes. Pizza was invented in Italy as a food for starving peasants and in Italy the poorer the region the thicker the pizza base. In Naples pizza was a very thick doughy base with a very simple tomato and cheese topping, it was a portable food for peasants working in the fields. Pizza was literally a plate made of dough on which to transport a worker's lunch. In Venice, where many wealthy Italians lived, the pizza base was very thin with much more elaborate meat and fish toppings.

In poor countries within their jails and mental institutions the diet is based around cereals purely because they are so cheap. It is (I know I keep repeating it because I want you to get it) cattle feed. Cereals are used to fatten cattle and when humans eat it, it fattens them too. Why would you eat cattle feed as your staple diet when you are free not to, when you have a choice? One of my clients who was in a mental hospital for months said that when he came out he could not look at bread and cereal ever again, because it reminded him of the bland hospital fare. I was in hospital briefly a few years ago and having had nothing at all to eat for twenty-four hours I was looking forward to some fruit or eggs for breakfast. I was offered only cereal, white toast and jam, they did not have any alternative so I chose to go without until I could have something that was more beneficial. When John McCarthy was freed from Lebanon he described his diet of pitta bread and cheese throughout his captivity. You have a choice to eat fish, fresh vegetables and salads with delicious dressing, grilled chicken and all kinds of fruits. Why are you eating like a pauper, a peasant, a prisoner when you have so many options? Even if you are very limited financially you can still eat well. In the long term it is cheaper to eat healthy fresh food than processed cereals.

If we think back to the diet of our ancestors, our grandparents did eat cereals but they were not refined or processed and they ate them alongside protein not instead of protein. They ate stews with vegetables and dumplings or meat with vegetables and potatoes. Most importantly they did not snack on convenience foods. Snack foods have been growing in popularity since the sixties and we have been growing fatter at an alarming rate as we eat them. Many of our grandparents were also expending a huge amount of physical energy as many jobs were more manual and consequently they were slimmer because of the sheer amount of energy used in manual labour. That is not the case anymore. Pasties were designed for miners to take down mines and sustain them throughout a long gruelling work shift, as were pies. I can understand a ploughman eating a ploughman's lunch to sustain him during a long farming day, but you and I do not need a huge hunk of glue stuffed with a huge hunk of mucus for the sedentary lifestyles we have nowadays.

Scotsmen would take dried porridge cut into squares or rolled into balls for a working lunch when they spent twelve hours in the fields. American farmers took hard-boiled eggs and dried grits (cold sliced porridge made of corn) to sustain them all day. They had a very bland diet with little variety and they ate much less in terms of amount than we do. This happens naturally when you limit the variety of food you eat. By limiting the variety of their meals our ancestors coped with food that is hard to digest. Also it was not full of pesticides, chemicals and preservatives.

The Western population has got bigger and fatter in direct proportion to the increase in cereal products being eaten as meals instead of accompaniments to meals and the addition of additives and convenience foods. A hundred years ago people ate much more healthy foods, they had less variety of food at each meal, they did more manual work and lived in homes without central heating which made them burn off more calories. Years ago we might have had some bread with a meal or a cake for afternoon tea, whereas now instead of having carbohydrates in addition to a meal the carbohydrates are the meal. Our grandparents and great grandparents did not eat rice, pasta, pizza, noodles, couscous, burritos, tacos, crisps, nachos, corn chips and pretzels. Sugar-laden breakfast cereals and cans of fizzy drink did not exist for them but now in addition to eating these things we also eat a full carbohydrate meal instead of anything else. This is linked to a staggering rise in weight. In some parts of the Western world over 70 per cent of the population are overweight.

Our bodies are designed to digest raw food, real food such as vegetables, fruits, nuts and seeds. These foods are easy to digest leaving our energy free to repair our bodies and eliminate toxins which are stored in fat cells. Eating dead, inert, processed and refined foods takes up so much valuable energy that our bodies have none left for other important tasks. Blood is diverted from our brain and organs to digest food and we fall asleep as a consequence. If you always fall asleep or feel sleepy after eating that is a sign you are eating the wrong food. If your stomach is flatter in the morning and distended by evening that is another sign, so is passing gas soon after eating. Your stomach is above your navel your intestines are below it. It is your intestines, your gut that swells due to distension. Your body does a good job of telling you what it doesn't like by reacting with heartburn, gas, skin eruptions, headaches, fatigue and bloating. If you listen to your body and work with it, listen to the messages your body is sending you and act on them, then you will begin looking and feeling different.

When I was at university I shared a flat with three other girls and we lived on really cheap food, mostly toast, bread, potatoes, pasta, cheese and cereal. We ate so badly that only when I had been living there for a year and my boyfriend brought over a chicken to cook did we discover the oven had never been connected, only the hob worked. Every night we would spend the whole evening sitting on the sofas watching TV, our jeans undone as our stomachs were so distended by the end of the day we could not sit comfortably.

Foods that originated as cereal are not only unhealthy because of the way they are processed, they can also be highly addictive for many people and disrupt, sometimes in an extreme way, our attempts to shed weight. In fact these very foods can cause our bodies to store excess fat. I will try to explain why as simply as possible. Refined and processed foods release large amounts of glucose very quickly causing a rapid rush in blood sugar followed by a rapid drop and consequently a craving for more of those foods. Blood sugar levels are believed to be one of the controllers of hunger and we know that protein cuts hunger very quickly. Processed foods are usually very low in protein and high in carbohydrate. There are some foods that cause our bodies to store excess fat and that lead to food cravings and even food addictions. It's a vicious circle because eating refined foods in response to the cravings causes weight gain.

One side effect of being overweight is an impairment of the hormone insulin's ability to correctly process fats and sugars. This impairment is called insulin resistance. Insulin resistance causes the body to store more fat than it needs to, especially around the middle. Hmm, is this reminding you of anyone yet, like you maybe? If the answer is yes then you are on the right track. You have to understand a problem to fix it. Adding to the problem, when your insulin levels rise due to an excess of carbohydrates, it sends your body a hormonal message telling it to store fat while holding on to the fat that's already there. So not only do excess carbohydrates make you fat, they keep you fat.

Eating a diet high in refined carbohydrates is the equivalent of eating two cups of pure table sugar a day. Since some starches such as white bread, white rice and potatoes increase blood sugar levels faster than table sugar, the food pyramid is encouraging us to consume sugar in large quantities as a healthy food. How could that possibly be healthy? White bread is so processed it is as bad for you as eating biscuits. In fact there is not much difference between white bread and white cake in nutritional content or the amount of carbohydrates and sugars. To make white bread all the bran and fibre are stripped away. One of the reasons why people who are wheat intolerant find white bread causes them less stomach discomfort and distension than brown bread is because so much is removed and the parts of the grain that are left are then pulverised milled and ground. In the baking process it becomes full of air. White bread is inert dead food of zero nutritional value. When it enters your bloodstream is has the same effect as eating three spoons of sugar. White bread is full of sugar. The more refined and preprocessed the food is the more it encourages weight gain. When sugar goes into your bloodstream too quickly your blood sugar surges, your pancreas overproduces insulin and you crave more carbohydrates the way an alcoholic craves alcohol. The excess sugar in your bloodstream gets stored in your fat cells.

Fast breakdown of sugars and starches into the bloodstream = Fast weight gain.

It really is as simple as that. If you want to lose weight and keep it off, eat real food and eat it slowly. Cutting out processed food will cut out the primary cause of excess weight. Anything that speeds up the digestion of carbohydrates can lead to weight gain. Anything that slows it down will help you to become and stay slim

It is becoming recognised that for many people refined carbohydrates are absolutely addictive. If this is the case for you then like an addict you have to cut them out of your life. You won't even miss them after a while. When you cut bad carbohydrates out of your diet you begin to reverse your body's inability to correctly process starches and sugar. This inability is the cause of most weight gain because it has such a disruptive effect on your blood chemistry. When your blood chemistry changes you will stop having cravings for the very foods that caused your excess weight.

Sugar, fat, salt and refined carbohydrates are highly addictive. Fruit, vegetables, nuts, seeds and protein are not addictive at all. Reading this book is systematically removing any painful thoughts you may have had about changing your diet and instead it is making you want to do it, ensuring you will like it, and feel good about it as the hypnotic content of this book is helping you implement powerful changes. The following exercise will reinforce your mind even more dramatically.

Grip Testing

1 To do this, put your thumb against your middle finger and push them together really, really hard while someone tries to pull and prise your finger and thumb apart. You should be able to resist very well.

2 Now hold a suspect item of food in your other hand – chocolate, white bread, cake or a biscuit and get the same person to try to prise apart the finger and thumb of the opposite hand while you push them together. You will find that your strength diminishes and your fingers can be pulled apart much more easily.

3 Now swap the bad food for something healthy like fruit or an avocado. Repeat the test and you will find that your grip strengthens as you hold healthy food in your hand.

4 Again to make this more powerful hold the item of food under your nose as you repeat stages 1, 2 and 3.

In doing this grip test you are proving to yourself again that your body knows the foods you should be avoiding. You lose all your strength when holding bad foods – your body has a negative reaction just holding them, let alone eating them.

This is a great exercise to do when you have children and want to teach them that some foods are bad for them. It is great fun to walk around a supermarket with your children and do 'the grip test' as they hold grapes or pears and again as they hold fizzy drinks, confectionery and crisps. In doing this you are making your children feel that they are making these choices rather than having them forced upon them by an overbearing parent.

Now that you have done these tests it does not mean you can't eat bread or pasta anymore, you can still eat them occasionally and still enjoy them too but recognise they are not a foods to be eaten all day and every day. The reason these tests are so important are that they prove to *you* what *your* body likes and dislikes. You are going to come up against people who say, 'Cereal is so healthy, bread is so good for you', I hear it all the time. Some of my relatives don't agree with my way of eating, and I have even been told 'Jesus ate bread'. Well, yes he did but it was made from spelt, a very healthy young sprouted seed that is nothing like modern wheat.

When I am doing interviews the interviewer often says to me, 'I don't have a problem with wheat so how can what you say be true?' My favourite reply is, 'Well, guess what? I don't have a problem with nuts or fish but if I meet people who do I don't say to them, "I don't have a reaction to nuts so you can't either", I accept that we have different bodies and different reactions to food.'

It's becoming more accepted by many healthcare professionals that overweight people generally can't digest wheat products or dairy very well and it makes them gain more weight and hampers their ability to shed weight. You don't need to prove this to anyone or to convert anyone, just do this for yourself.

Keeping It Off Forever

Time For Action – Simple Steps, Massive Results

This is one major step that contains many small steps that will give you fantastic and lifelong results. If you want to look different you have to *do* different and it has to be all the time; dieting to lose weight then resuming the habits that got you overweight is pointless. We don't just want to drop weight for a short while, we want to keep it off forever, and these steps will enable you to keep off the weight you have shed. At this very important stage of the book you have replaced many habits of thought that got you overweight and now you are ready to replace some actions that also got you overweight. This time you are doing it the right way round, replacing the negative thoughts and then replacing the negative actions.

Ten Actions to Keep It Off For Good

1. TO CHANGE WHAT GOES INTO YOU, CHANGE WHAT YOU KEEP IN THE HOUSE

One of the most important changes you can make is changing what you keep in your house. If you go into the kitchen of a celebrity or anyone who successfully controls their weight you will find they are as disciplined about what they keep in their house as they are about what they eat. Sometimes if I am working late, writing through the night, I know that if I had a big bag of nachos in the house I would eat them, but since I don't I can't. I can only snack on healthy food because I do not have an alternative to hand. Since I don't have biscuits around I snack on tinned pineapple or berries instead.

You can stop buying junk food, sweets, biscuits, crisps and chocolate. You don't need to keep them for visitors or for your children. Give your children money to buy themselves treats but do not have tempting things in your house. If they are not there you can't eat them. Throw them all away and don't replace them. If I do buy biscuits for my daughter I deliberately buy the ones I don't like, the same with ice cream and crisps. It is so much easier for me to avoid them this way.

Your kids will thank you for not surrounding them with junk as you will be teaching them not to eat it and ensuring they do not grow up addicted to junk foods with the accompanying disrupted blood chemistry. You are doing them a favour, helping them for life and being a good parent by denying them high-calorie, low-nutrient foods. Of course, they won't thank you immediately, but they will later. I have never denied my daughter sweets but she has to go out and get them. I have also never made her finish food and she has a really healthy relationship with food and therefore won't ever be overweight. She takes a little then goes back for more and she leaves food when she's had enough. I work with many overweight children and it is heartbreaking to hear of how they feel inadequate and are bullied and diminished because of their weight. You can still allow your children ice cream, cakes and crisps and sweets, but if they are not kept in the house they will get eaten a lot less.

So many people I work with buy junk for their partners and children and eat it all themselves. The excuse that they are buying it for others is redundant. If you keep junk food in the house for your children and they end up with the same weight problem as you then you have not done them any favours. People who have stopped drinking don't keep alcohol in the house for other people, and people who have quit smoking don't have a packet of cigarettes on the coffee table, just in case a guest might like one, they banish the items that were their weaknesses. My friends who are vegans would never have animal protein in the house and when I go to their house for dinner I eat what they eat.

You need to be organised about buying the right food, buying enough of it and always having it to hand otherwise you will give in to temptation. Keep the right foods in your cupboard and fridge and buy good alternatives to the things you used to crave. I always have tinned, dried and fresh pineapple as it works for me when I crave something sweet and it contains a natural digestive enzyme. I buy bags of frozen prawns three at a time so I can make a prawn and tomato omelette in minutes if I come home really hungry. Years ago I would have made cheese on toast or eaten biscuits but those days are long gone and never missed.

By following the suggestions for ideal fridge and pantry staples in this book you will always have the right foods to hand. Eating badly creates such a vicious circle that you may not feel you have the energy to stock up. However, buying and eating the correct foods will give you so much more energy. We all have to shop, so just shop more effectively and banish the wrong foodstuffs from your home.

2. LIMIT VARIETY

Another very important step is limiting the variety of food you eat at each meal. We need to eat a varied diet but too much variety at mealtimes causes overeating which causes weight gain. We should have a variety of healthy food over a period of each day but have less variety at every meal. Less is more. Too much variety makes us fat because we gain weight when our appetite drives us to eat too much, so we don't know when to stop, especially when faced with masses of variety at all-you-can-eat buffets or parties and functions with lots of varieties of food.

Appetite is created by five triggers:

1 Production of stomach acid.
2 An empty stomach.
3 Sight and smell of food.
4 Action of the appetite centre in the hypothalamus area of the brain.
5 Conditioned reflex – eating even if we are not hungry just because its a mealtime or food is in front of us.

This last point happens on long-haul flights. I fly to America frequently and on the flight the airline serves afternoon tea at 4 p.m. local time when for everyone on the plane it is 2 a.m. which really isn't the kind of time we would want afternoon tea, and on the return flight they wake us at 4 a.m. London time to serve breakfast. If we had to pay for these meals we would pass on them but because they are free and put in front of us they get eaten.

Constant overeating stretches the stomach wall so that it takes longer to feel full. Your stomach will shrink back when you consistently eat less.

We overeat junk food when our appetite is overstimulated with taste enhancers and chemicals, and when our senses are overstimulated with too much choice. All humans have an inbuilt 'sensory specific satiety' which means there is only so much of one food we can eat before we get bored and naturally stop eating. This innate appetite control is overridden by variety and newness in textures and flavours which is why we can be absolutely full after a big Sunday lunch but still get tempted by the desserts. You know how it is when we are in a restaurant and say, 'I couldn't eat another thing, I am absolutely stuffed' and then the desserts come out and we are tempted by something different, a new taste, texture and flavour. Limiting the variety of food available naturally limits our intake of food and keeps us slimmer.

All animals have natural satiety and will stop eating after a while but when we give them our food then they will overeat and become fat. This happens when we give domestic pets sweets, cakes and other food they could not get if they were hunting for it themselves. It also happens when laboratory animals are fed processed food and it happens in zoos when the animals are given too much variety.

When are we faced with too much variety? At a breakfast buffet, for instance, with ten varieties of bread, muffins and pastries. Eggs cooked in five different ways, a table full of every kind of breakfast cereal, every kind of jam, fruit, dried fruit and bacon, sausage, mushroom, tomatoes and potatoes. We are easily tempted to take far too much and to try a little of everything and we end up overfull, bloated and lacking energy. Even at home if you made a breakfast of scrambled eggs with mushrooms you would eat less than if you had bacon, eggs, mushrooms, beans, tomatoes and toast. Your taste buds would not be so stimulated by too much variety which would not encourage you to overeat.

I stayed at a hotel in Dubai and the evening buffet was so vast it was spread over three different rooms. They had dishes from almost every country and another separate area just to house all the desserts. Most people overate because it was a set price no matter how much you ate or how many times you returned for more, and the food was so tempting and so varied you had to overeat if you wanted to sample all of it.

We overeat on junk, stodge and sweets much more than we would on, say, unlimited chicken or unlimited eggs. We become satisfied and less hungry on protein and stop eating quite quickly when we eat basic protein. The amino acids in protein send a message of fullness to our brains rapidly. Protein changes the biochemistry in our brain because protein-rich foods encourage the production of the hormone peptide YY which is known to suppress appetite.

If we were eating a whole chicken it's unlikely we would finish it, or a whole pan of soup or lamb stew. Even with confectionery, when we have a box of assorted chocolates or fancy biscuits we want to try them all but if they are all the same we are less likely to finish the box. If you had a big box of plain digestive biscuits you probably wouldn't finish it but when you have assorted biscuits even as you eat the bourbon you are planning to eat the custard cream then the jammie dodger then the chocolate digestive and so on. If you think of the variety involved in Christmas lunch it's no wonder people fall asleep in front of the TV afterwards and report weight gain over the holidays. Originally, the Victorian Christmas lunch consisted of turkey, parsnips, potatoes, sprouts and carrots. Now it also includes stuffing, sausages wrapped in bacon, bread sauce, Christmas cake, Christmas pudding, trifle, mince pies, endless chocolates and alcohol. We can love and enjoy Christmas lunch but still limit the amount and variety of food we eat and avoid the processed foods as there are so many other foods to enjoy.

In order to control conditioned reflex eating, treat all-you-can-eat buffets with caution. If you are eating at a buffet go up and be selective in serving yourself, aiming for protein and vegetables and filling your plate to what you think is a reasonable portion for a meal, but not too much. *And do not return for more.* Do not delude yourself that you must eat it because it's free and remember that you already served yourself a full-sized portion so why would you need more? The notion of eating more because it's free is a lie. I have clients who would frequent all-you-can-eat establishments and then spend hundreds even thousands of pounds trying various quick fixes, miracle diets, pills, liposuction and gym memberships to work off the excess fat. They spent much more trying to get rid of the weight than they ever saved in gaining it.

I love that expression, 'Take whatever you want and then pay for it.' It's an old Jewish saying but it could have been written for the all-you-can-eat restaurants. My other favourite saying is, 'If you are not part of the solution you are part of the problem.' Be a part of the solution. Don't have too much variety at each meal and don't keep the wrong foods in your house.

3. STOP EATING CARBS AFTER LUNCH

One of the keys to weight loss is to eat some protein at every meal and to eat healthy carbohydrates such as fruits and vegetables, but to eat far fewer bad carbohydrates such as bread, potatoes and pasta. In the previous chapter I explained how detrimental these foods are for people with weight issues but only you can decide whether to keep them in your diet or not. If you love them and cannot be without them then eat them at lunch but stop all cereals after your midday meal. Cereal is not just what you have for breakfast, it is everything made from grains including bread, pasta, pizza, pies and crackers (and it also includes rice).

On *Celebrity Fit Club*, when the contestants wanted to improve their weekly weight loss, they stopped eating bread, potatoes, pasta and rice after midday. You can even stop them after breakfast, it is quite safe and you will certainly drop weight by doing this.

If you do eat cereals at lunchtime you can make smarter choices such as brown rice with tuna instead of sandwiches, microwaved poppadoms are great too, gluten free and usually made with gram flour (lentil flour: lentils are pulses, not cereals). If you must have a sandwich, have it in the form of a wrap, a tortilla or brown pitta. Tortillas and pittas have much less dough than baguettes, rolls, bagels and French bread. It's so easy to resume eating cereals and to forget how much you've consumed and to increase their intake without really noticing it. Stopping cereals after lunch naturally restricts your intake of them without you feeling deprived. It allows you to stick to an easy routine without allowing your cereal intake to creep back up.

Rye, maize, millet, rice and barley are all cereals, but are much more digestible than wheat so eating rye bread and Ryvita instead of wheat bread or eating rice cakes is a better alternative if you are still eating cereals. When I was a child I used to feed my guinea pigs bran and my father would buy huge sacks of it for about twenty pence. It was only available in pet shops, no food shops sold it as it was not considered a food for human consumption. We would never have considered eating it any more than we would have considered eating the hay that was used to feed horses. Then it became marketed as a food to alleviate constipation and became fashionable and highly promoted despite it being too rough and corrosive for most people's intestines. I do not believe eating lots of glue makes people regular, but flaxseeds are a brilliant alternative for constipation. Flaxseeds are also known as linseeds – only buy the milled flaxseeds or linseeds. They are a wonder food full of Omega oils and they are also excellent for your skin. Fruit and vegetables and enough water are usually sufficient to make you regular. If not have about three teaspoons of flaxseeds every other day and you will be fine. They're easy to eat by adding them to smoothies, salads, soups or just sprinkle them into a small glass of water and drink them, they have no taste at all.

Of course, if you get invited out to a pasta dinner you can still participate. My programme is not rigid – it's flexible and adaptable – but do adhere to these rules most of the time in order to keep any excess weight off.

4. LIMIT LATE-NIGHT EATING

The next very simple step to keep excess weight off is not to eat late at night. Our bodies are simply not designed to have a big dinner at 10.30 p.m. and then go to bed. This is fine occasionally and, of course, you will still want to go out to dinner, but avoid eating late on a regular basis and try to make it as early as possible and never eat a snack before going to bed. Our bodies are still like those of caveman really since it takes hundreds of years to evolve and adapt. Primitive man got up with the light and retired as it got dark as there was nothing else to do. Eating too much and too late at night leaves our bodies full of undigested food. Our metabolism slows down dramatically at night even if we are wide awake, because nature assumes we're sleeping and therefore not as active as when we're awake so our heart-rate slows right down making digestion more difficult.

Going to bed on a full stomach means your body is working all night to digest food when it should be resting and as a result you are likely to wake up feeling tired rather that refreshed and with a food hangover. This is because at around 2 a.m. our bodies begin the cycle of cell repair essential to good health. The later it is in the evening the less we should eat since the cycle of cell repair is set aside when we go to bed on a full stomach because the same pancreatic enzymes used for cell repair are used for digestion. If you eat late all the time you will age much more rapidly and be more susceptible to illness and poor health because this process of cell repair will be put on hold as you digest food. The tiredness you feel in the morning may cause you to eat a sugary snack for a quick energy boost thus perpetuating a damaging eating pattern.

We are designed to sleep more and eat less and since electricity was invented humans have increasingly slept less and eaten more and are suffering because of it. If you do find yourself eating too late at night because of social or work issues you could help your body's digestion process by taking natural digestive enzymes after your meal which you can buy in a health food shop. They will help your body break down the food.

Remember, the human body has a cycle of its own. It digests food best during the day, the earlier the better, and digests food very poorly at night. The body conducts all its detoxifying work between 11 p.m. and 2 a.m. So if you go to bed after 2 a.m. you may wake up feeling as tired as if you hadn't slept. It's good to go to bed hungry as it means you are burning off fat and you can have a healthy breakfast in the morning. Since eating is supposed to give us energy there is no benefit at all in a late-night snack we don't need the energy since we are about to sleep.

5. FAST FOOD MAKES YOU FAT FAST.

This next step is one you have heard over and over: avoid fast food.

It isn't a coincidence that the fattest nations eat the most fast food. Eating fast food once a day means you are eating up to one pound of sugar daily and 1,700 calories in one meal – almost a full day's allowance. The danger with fast food is not just the fact that it is cooked really fast in saturated fat that is often rancid, but that it is eaten so fast. Fast food is given that name because it's so quick to prepare and even quicker to consume. Burgers, chips, doughnuts, sandwiches and pizza are very easy to bolt down in a matter of minutes. Because this food is nutritionally very poor we are likely to be hungry again far too quickly. Our body will continue to demand food because it is not getting any nutrients from the junk food we have put into it.

Fast food is often full of taste enhancers which need to be avoided as they are chemicals designed to make you crave more and therefore overeat. Fast food restaurants also load their food with chemicals which make the food break down in your mouth really quickly like baby food. We love food that breaks down quickly. Think of chocolate and how it melts on your tongue immediately. Butter, cream, ice cream, cakes and creamy desserts, buttered popcorn, hot white toast and butter require no effort to break down in your mouth. We eat too much of these types of foods because it's so easy. This is because your appetite is stimulated yet your brain is not registering that you are eating because you are eating too quickly. The only reason the fast food industry alters its food with taste enhancers is because we consume more of it. When you can wolf down a burger in minutes you will buy another one.

It's a money-making venture. When we eat quickly our stomach doesn't even register that it's full until twenty minutes later. Real food like vegetables or a grilled steak require a lot of chewing to break them down so we feel full and satisfied much sooner.

Research by American scientists suggests fat and sugar in high quantities have a similar effect on the brain as opiates and cocaine, which means that we get high on the chemicals in processed foods. Remember how cheese protein has opiates in it and is highly addictive. High-fat chemical-laden snacks like crisps can affect the liver and gall bladder and are addictive. Doctors have discovered that the drug-like effects certain foods have on our brain is very similar to alcohol and keeps us wanting more, and because this kind of food is so easily and quickly consumed we're not aware of how much we've eaten, which means that most overweight people do overeat although many think they don't. The very food we should not eat is chemically altered to make us want it all the time and in large quantities. Do you recall the advert that said 'Bet you can't eat just one'. Of course you can't eat just one, it's been chemically altered to ensure you eat several. Advertisers know this and play on it – this is what you are up against when you eat chemically altered food. If someone pointed out to you that a particular food was highly addictive and proven to not only cause tremendous weight gain but also to make you want even more of it in the process and to make you ill, unhealthy and very unhappy, why would you continue to eat it when there are many lovely alternatives available to replace it? *This book is that someone.*

When we become addicted to a food and eat it all the time and in excessive amounts our bodies are likely to become intolerant and sensitive to that food. The symptoms of the intolerance will show as headaches, irritable bowel syndrome, indigestion, bad skin, tiredness, weight gain and difficulty sustaining weight reduction. The common symptoms of eating badly are that body fat increases, your liver becomes fatty and you may get frequent headaches. High-fat fast food is extremely harmful to your heart, liver and blood, in fact it can be as dangerous to your liver as alcohol.

If you accept that these foods are addictive and promoted by companies who want to keep you addicted to their products because of the vast profit involved you can then choose to break the pattern of addiction and overeating. Remember earlier in the book when I asked you to work out how long you could feel good for after eating junk food? For most people it's only minutes and even if you could feel good for an hour after eating junk it's still never worth it – remembering that helps you to change.

Another reason to avoid fast food is that the incidence of diabetes is rising in the West and its rise is linked to eating fast food. A new medical study shows that eating in fast food restaurants more than twice a week increases the risk of diabetes because it increases insulin resistance. Syndrome X, a pre-diabetic condition that leaves sufferers feeling lethargic and generally unwell, is also rising dramatically. Syndrome X happens when blood cells become overrun with sugars and can no longer burn off enough of the sugar, so it becomes stored as fat instead. Fast food is full of sugar and it's easy to eat too much sugar as it doesn't fill us up.

The message about the damaging effects of fast food is finally hitting home because many fast food restaurants are trying to reverse some of their negative publicity by promoting salads. However, some McDonald's salads are loaded with sugar and fat in the dressings and are just as high in calories as a burger. It's also worth noting that Ben Cohen of Ben and Jerry's Ice Cream had triple bypass surgery at the age of forty-three. The founder of Baskin Robbins had diabetes at an early age while his brother who worked alongside him in the ice cream industry died of a heart attack at sixty.

Try a different kind of fast food. Some of my favourite dishes are cooked fast; scrambled eggs, omelettes, stir-fried vegetables, seared tuna, grilled fish, stir fried chicken or turkey fillets are all dishes that can be cooked in minutes but they are healthy and will not lead to weight gain.

You have to take this eating plan seriously. Saying, 'Oh they only had pizza so I had no choice but to eat it' is an excuse. A vegan or Muslim would never say, 'I had to eat the pork, it was all that was available and I didn't want to hurt their feelings'. Nuts, fruit and seeds are nature's portable food. I always carry unsalted almonds, pumpkin seeds and fruit when I am travelling. J Lo or Madonna would never eat cake because nothing else was available. They put themselves first and make sure what they want is available. When Princess Diana visited everyday people in their homes she would have a member of her staff call them in advance to let them know that she liked to be served bananas, pears and black coffee. This was food that she liked, that was inexpensive and always available so her hosts could always provide it without anyone feeling embarrassed. She also ensured that her staff always carried some healthy food that she could eat and would not eat cakes or pastries just because they were offered. She was frequently given homemade cakes and boxes of chocolates by people who had gone to a lot of effort to make them for her and she always accepted them very graciously saying that she would have them later or save them for her boys or ladies in waiting. You don't need to be a princess to do the same thing, you can graciously accept food that is offered but you don't have to eat it and you can graciously decline it.

You must make your needs more important than those of your host. Your need to be slim, healthy and live a long life has to be more important than your need to please someone else. Some of my clients can't even ask a waiter they don't know and will never see again to prepare their food differently. Those in the food service industry will accommodate your needs if you ask them nicely and appreciate their efforts. At other people's homes as long as you refuse food graciously and ask for something simple like some eggs or even offer something you have with you nobody will mind. Eat like a star, like a celebrity. Movie stars and athletes have no problem requesting special food because they know they are worth it, that they will get it and it is important to them. Making it important is the same belief that allows people with allergies or religious needs to ask for different food. Do you think Brad Pitt or David Beckham can't ask for special food? Celebrities are not embarrassed about being different in fact they like being different, they know they are worth it. You are worth it too.

Wheat flour does not agree with me but I don't tell anyone it makes me gain weight like a sumo wrestler because I always get back comments like, 'Oh one little bit won't hurt' or, 'You could do with gaining weight' or, 'Well go on a diet tomorrow I made it especially' or, 'Just taste it, have a little to please me', 'This is organic healthy flour you will like it'. When you say, 'Wheat makes me ill and gives me chronic headaches' you will get a much more sympathetic reaction. No one is going to reply, 'So what, just stay in bed all day tomorrow and take medication' or, 'I have some painkillers in the bathroom why don't you have some for later'. If you said I have a dangerous reaction to nuts you will not hear back 'Oh go on, it's only one, who cares if you go into anaphylactic shock later?'

As a Muslim, Jew, Buddhist, Sikh or Rastafarian you would refuse certain foods because of your religious beliefs and your needs would be respected and accommodated, likewise as a vegetarian or a diabetic. But if you feel uncomfortable refusing food because you are on a programme to shed weight I totally understand that it can feel awkward making special requests and being selective about what you will or won't eat. The easiest solution is to just say, 'It does not agree with me and makes me really unwell'. You will be telling the truth, if you are overweight or have had a lifelong issue with weight I would put money on the fact that the wrong foods are part if not all of the cause. Always remind yourself of how important you are.

One of the major contributory factors to gaining weight is that people eat on the run, they snack all the time. Over 50 per cent of the calories in our diets come from snack food and junk food. My own research found that people break their diets when they are too tired to wait to eat so they grab sugary snacks or the nearest available food or anything to boost their flagging energy. When people are on the move or out and about and don't have access to the foods on their exclusion or restriction diet they will eat anything. Not you though, you will break the vicious circle of being tired from eating indigestible nutritionally empty food when you have the right foods available to you all the time. Having portable food with you will smash the negative pattern and free you from the vicious cycle while giving you the energy to live your life. You must get into the habit of having some of the right food with you and once you start to do this it becomes second nature.

When my daughter was a baby I would never have left the house without my baby bag that contained food and drinks for her. I could not stop at a garage and buy her a snack so I took the things she needed with me everywhere I went. All mothers do this – go to any park and you will see them unpacking food for the baby and snacks for the toddlers. It would be inconceivable not to do that and because it's necessary it simply becomes part of a mother's routine. Get into the same routine of carrying some foods for you, simple portable things like fruit and nuts. I have clients who even carry a snack and a bottle of water for their dog but think it is too much work to carry food for themselves.

One in four people visiting their doctor report being tired all the time and this is mostly caused by a poor diet or the wrong diet for that person. Diet books promote eating three healthy meals a day around the table and while this is a wonderful ideal it just is not going to happen for everyone. I have clients who never cook and instead they only ever heat food up or buy ready meals and take outs. The amount of convenience food on sale nowadays shows what a burgeoning market it has become and how the number of people who don't cook has increased. People working ten to fourteen hours a day are not going to start preparing and cooking food unless it is quick. Indeed, recent studies show that a third of Britons never cook at all. Rather than insisting on a total change, this book works with your way of life. This section will show you how to snack and still lose weight and stay healthy by eating instant healthy food. My clients love my advice on portable foods and what food items to have in your fridge, pantry and freezer. We need to get into a lifelong habit of having the right food in our car, bag, office, desk, locker or travel bag etc., as well as having the right food at home. They all tell me this was life changing for them. Having the right food to hand, having the right food at home, having it in bulk and having healthy food they could prepare in minutes. We assume people know how to eat and how to shop when in fact they often don't, hence a resulting weight problem. Guidelines are very useful in resolving weight issues but they need to be suited to your life on a long-term basis, which is why diets work for a limited time only and are too restricting to stay with long term.

So, if you want to keep the weight off and look and feel fabulous you need to buy portable food and always have it to hand. Make sure you bulk buy raw (unsalted and unsmoked) almonds and tins of ring-pull tuna, crab, salmon, sardines and mackerel. When you are rushing out of the door it's so easy to grab a can of fish, some cherry tomatoes, an avocado and some fruit and nuts and you have something very healthy and sustaining to eat. It may not be the best food you have ever eaten but if your alternative is prepackaged sandwiches and a packet of crisps you have already made a massive improvement. If you keep nuts and canned fish (you can also buy tuna and salmon in foil pouches) in your car and keep some canned fish, some nuts and seeds, fruit and cartons of soya milk and soya yogurt (long life obviously) in your desk or locker at work you will always have something to eat in an emergency situation.

It's a good idea to take some foodstuff along these lines when you are travelling. Recently on a flight I wanted to buy something to eat but ended up buying nothing as all the airline had to sell were crisps, chocolates, sandwiches, muffins and fizzy drinks. Trains are not much better, their staple fare is pizza, sandwiches, burgers, biscuits and crisps because there is so much profit to be made selling these foods and they don't have to worry about their shelf life. As this type of junk food seems to be the norm, it's much safer to take your own healthy alternatives. I am amazed at how many of my clients say they would be too embarrassed to eat their own food in public but would not be embarrassed to eat jumbo bags of crisps and bars of chocolate even when they are overweight. You can take a Tupperware of chicken or tuna salad on a flight or train but if you are too self conscious some nuts, seeds and fruit will sustain you until you can eat proper food.

I always carry food with me because carrying my own food means I can eat what I want when I want to. If I am out and I get hungry I will buy a packet of prawns or chicken and eat it wherever I am. I have often done this in supermarkets rather than buy chocolate or cakes. It doesn't look any worse than walking round a store eating crisps, and if you're worried about any mess then just buy baby wipes for your fingers afterwards. I keep a carrier bag in my car that always has in it some unsalted almonds, some mixed seeds, some foil pouches of fish and a packet of sun-dried tomatoes and some small cartons of rice milk. When I am rushing out of the house and may be gone all day it's so easy to grab some fruit like an apple, a pear and a banana and maybe an avocado or box of cherry tomatoes and add them to my bag then I know I have enough food to last me all day wherever I am.

I was lecturing in a barn in the middle of nowhere last year and the caterer didn't show up so the host sent out for pizzas. I was so glad I could make myself something I love to eat from my bag. I hate pizza – it gives me indigestion and makes me want to go to sleep soon after eating it and since I had to lecture all afternoon I needed to be alert. I don't care about being different – I care much more about looking and feeling healthy and I never make a big deal of it so no one takes much notice at all. I have frequently been in meetings that have overrun so sandwiches are brought in or been on film sets where the host has made a huge bowl of pasta for us or gone to dinner parties where pasta is the only thing on the menu. Because I always have some canned fish in the car I just ask them if I can have that with some nuts or salad. No one has ever minded because I ask nicely and explain that wheat flour makes me ill. Without making a fuss you can say I'm sorry but wheat gives me the most dreadful headaches, it looks so delicious but I can't risk it so could I have a tin of tuna fish and a bit of salad or some eggs instead? As long as you refuse food graciously and ask for something simple like some eggs or even offer something you have with you it will be fine. At a restaurant you will have some choices. If you are going to a dinner party it is fine to phone ahead to tell your host you cannot eat wheat flour while offering to bring something to eat or share.

I have sat in meetings pulling the bread away from sandwiches and eating only the filling. Vegetarians would pull out the filling if it was meat and eat just the bread and no one really cares. Even in sandwich bars I just ask for a selection of the fillings. In pizza restaurants I do the same, I just enjoy a variety of the toppings. I would much rather feel a little different than be overweight and I'm sure you would too. I have been both and I know a little inconvenience is much easier to live with than being fat. Waiters don't mind at all as long as you are polite and appreciative. Even if I was in a fish and chip shop I would order just fish and get them to take the batter off the fish or do it myself. I have been able to do this in the most challenging situations like being on the road all week or touring Italy and Cornwall with my family, and it really is easy once you know it's the right thing for you.

8. PANTRY STAPLES

Taking this programme seriously means thinking ahead and preparing. Be your own PA and make sure you have the right foods in your fridge or in your bag. You have to have the correct foods in your fridge and pantry and you have to have the incorrect foods gone. It is no good buying one can of fish and one bag of nuts and seeds. You need to buy ten packets of nuts and seeds and ten cans of fish. I am amazed when I tell my patients how to eat and they say, 'Well I took your advice and I bought a packet of prawns and some nuts but then I ran out of them so I had to eat the biscuits instead'. Take it seriously and buy your essential items in triplicate so that you never run out of anything.

Always have a box of organic eggs to hand and some frozen prawns so you can make a prawn omelette in minutes, you can add frozen spinach or sweet corn too. Have some precooked frozen dishes like chicken casserole or a stew in the freezer so you can make a meal very quickly when you are hungry. Sometimes I just open a tin of tuna or salmon and eat it with an avocado and some tomatoes and sweet corn. It takes seconds to put together and is filling and nutritious. If your weakness is reaching for food when you come home and not being able to wait to eat, then have a bowl of hard-boiled eggs shelled and ready so that you can snack on two hard boiled eggs, some tomatoes, lettuce and a little dressing. It is delicious, will cut your hunger within twenty minutes and takes only two minutes more than it does to reach for the biscuits (you don't have biscuits in your house anymore, right?)

In place of biscuits buy some nut and seed bars (you must check they are free of flour and sugar). My favourites are by the Food Doctor and Gillian McKeith. You can make your own mixture of nuts and seeds but do not buy ready-made trail mix since it's full of sugar.

9. NOT ALL FAT MAKES YOU FAT

You don't need to exclude fat; good fats are healthy and vital for our wellbeing. Essential fatty acids found in nuts, fish and avocado actually cleanse the body of the saturated fats that make the blood sticky. Avocado is one of the healthiest foods in the world. Lean meat is not bad for you. Oily fish is an excellent food. Fats have more calories than carbohydrates but are *not* more fattening. When we eat healthy fats we become satisfied quickly, whereas when we eat refined carbohydrates we are actually stimulated to overeat because their effect on our blood sugar leaves us constantly hungry. We have been taught to see fat as a baddie, the cause of obesity and heart attacks, yet Mediterranean people eat diets rich in olive oil. Olive oil is a good fat, as are fish oils, nut oils, vegetable oils and seed oils such as sunflower, pumpkin and hemp, which are full of essential fatty acids. Even animal fat (saturated) is not bad as long as it is eaten in moderation.

Nuts are one of nature's wonder foods; buy raw almonds, pistachios, walnuts, hazelnuts. Brazil nuts are an excellent source of selenium which is a cancer preventative food. Selenium reduces the amount of mercury the body absorbs and is recommended if you eat a lot of fish. Nuts are not especially fattening since the oil in them is not fully absorbed by the body. Not all the fat and therefore not all the calories of nuts are absorbed as some of the fat is bound up with fibre and passes out of the body. Nuts are very filling and help build strong bones and they contain good healthy oils rich in mono and polyunsaturated fats that help prevent heart attacks. Always keep your nuts and seeds in containers in the fridge to stop the oils going rancid.

I have always believed eggs are a wonder food and new research is backing this up. Free-range organic eggs are very good for you as they contain vitamin A, B, D and E and lutein which protects against age-related eye diseases. Furthermore, eggs are less chemically altered than most other foods. Eggs are rich in lecithin and although the yolks contain cholesterol they will not raise cholesterol levels in the blood unless you have an inherited cholesterol problem. It is the saturated fats in food not natural dietary cholesterol that raises blood cholesterol levels. As long as the eggs you eat form part of a balanced diet you can eat far more than the previous guideline of five a week.

People get very confused about good and bad foods I call good foods 'growing foods' i.e. vegetables, salads, nuts, seeds and fruits. Foods that can be picked and eaten exactly as they are without anything needing to be done to them can be eaten freely. Fruit juice is not in this category as it has to be juiced, pressed or concentrated. Primitive man may have eaten a few oranges or apples but drinking juice allows us to eat the equivalent of ten oranges in one go without the healthy fibre and pulp so we get a huge sugar rush and then crave more sugar in any form throughout the day. Eat fruit rather than drinking juice.

Food that has to be milled and cooked like grains (including rice) are not in this category. These can be eaten in limited amounts but you need to choose brown rice, wholewheat granary or rye bread and wholewheat pasta. Orgran is pasta made from vegetables that you can buy in all large supermarkets and it is delicious. Rye, millet and barley are all cereals and while they are better for us than wheat they still need to be eaten moderately by those of us with a weight problem.

10. TRAIN YOUR APPETITE AND CUT CRAVINGS

Interestingly, we start to like what we eat the most of and want what our bodies get used to. Hence third generation Polish, Portuguese or Spaniards living in England still eat the diet they were primarily raised on, while vegetarians crave vegetables and people who live on fast food crave fast food. Since you will adapt to whatever you eat and find that eventually you only desire that type of food you might as well make your body love and crave healthy food. If you love sugar or full-fat milk in your tea and then give it up, after some time you will find that if you try it again it tastes horrible. When you abstain from fatty food it really does taste too greasy if you have it again after a long absence. After abstaining from sugary food it really does become far too sweet to enjoy except in small amounts. I eat chips with my daughter occasionally but only a few as I don't have any desire to eat more, and although I enjoy chips I wouldn't eat them regularly. I would always have mince pies at Christmas but I don't crave them and I'm happy to eat far fewer of them than I used to.

I was a vegetarian while I lived in California (and I still think being a vegetarian is a noble thing to do) and I thought I was so healthy. My diet included masses of vegetables, rice, potatoes and bread but I was always tired and very pale. By the end of the day my stomach was always bloated and I was hungry again shortly after eating. I would have bread and honey for breakfast, vegetables and rice for lunch and in the evening a huge plate of vegetables and potatoes. I snacked on muesli bars or crackers and I would want to eat every few hours. It was a huge revelation for me when one day after doing lots of research on protein and hunger I had chicken and vegetables for dinner and felt full and satisfied until the next day. As I put more protein in my diet and took out a lot of the cereals I felt so much more energetic, my whole shape changed dramatically and I shed a stone without even trying to.

Protein foods, like chicken, fish, lean meat, tofu and eggs stimulate the get-up-and-go brain chemicals called catecholamines that give you energy and leave you feeling satisfied and slim, not bloated, sleepy and still hungry. Protein is the only food that cuts hunger very quickly by sending a message of fullness to the brain. Just a small amount of protein will give you drive, energy and mental focus. The amino acids in protein tell our brain that we are full and affect appetite regulation in the brain in a way that carbohydrate foods don't.

Protein-rich foods encourage the production of the hormone peptide YY which is known to suppress appetite. You do not need to eat a lot of protein, a small amount at every meal is enough. For instance ten almonds added to fruit at breakfast is enough protein, a handful of nuts and seeds added to a salad at lunch, or a palm-sized amount of chicken or fish is all the protein you need, and you do need protein if you want to be slimmer. Of course you can have more than that amount if you find it doesn't satisfy you.

A Day in the Life of the New Thin You

So here you are at step ten having learned so much and come so far. By now I hope you agree that the small amount of time you have taken to read this book and do the exercises has been absolutely worthwhile. In this last chapter I am going to show you fifteen ways to speed up your metabolism. Again you don't have to do all fifteen, this is a pick and mix that makes you thinner, it's up to you which of them you choose, though of course the more of them you use the more impact you'll have in shifting excess weight and keeping it off. By incorporating these small changes into your life you can create big changes in your weight and shape.

You are also going to learn a new kind of takeaway – one that has no calories. These new takeaways summarise everything you have learned and show you how to make them a part of your daily life. There is no jargon, no deprivation and no gimmicks just practical step-by-step solutions that give you lasting results. These final few steps make it easy for you to put everything into practice. By embracing these new takeaways you will find it straightforward and simple to implement these powerful, beneficial and workable changes into your life and to change your shape forever.

Fifteen Ways to Rev Up Your Metabolism

Your metabolism determines the rate at which you burn calories and fat. The faster your metabolism the more fuel you will burn off.

VISUALISE

Since every thought you think causes a physical reaction in your body, if you frequently visualise your metabolism going up you can increase it. You need to constantly imagine your metabolism as a dial you are turning up to maximum and leaving it on maximum all the time. Imagine an internal furnace or heat within you burning off any excess fuel. Tell yourself your metabolism is super efficient and working at maximum efficiency all the time.

EAT REGULARLY

Eating pushes up your metabolic rate as digestion uses up calories. A lot of energy is consumed in the digestion process, as your gut contracts enzymes are released and extra blood is pumped to your intestines. If you don't eat regularly your metabolic rate goes down. Missing out on one meal a day will diminish your metabolism by 15 per cent. You will shed more weight eating selectively than you will by fasting.

GET ENOUGH SLEEP

Five hours or more of unbroken sleep helps your body to maintain balanced hormone levels related to metabolism. Sleep deprivation can produce a hormonal imbalance that can stimulate weight gain.

EXERCISE

Exercise will speed up your metabolism. If you are overweight you can still exercise. I am a big fan of rebounding – jumping on a mini trampoline. It takes only ten minutes a day and that time will fly by if you put on some great music. Because it is aerodynamic (low impact) your joints are protected. Skipping is also a quick and very effective exercise and at any weight you can skip for a few minutes and gradually build up the amount of time. I take a skipping rope away with me so I can do just a few minutes in my hotel room to keep my metabolic rate up. A group of inactive women put on a mini trampoline by James White, a Californian exercise physiologist, were monitored and found to have improvement in skin tone, colouring and wrinkles. Even the bags under their eyes decreased because the intense rhythmic pressure and the weightlessness of rebounding stimulate cells to release waste. As you become slimmer and fitter you may feel more ready to join a gym or class. You don't need me to tell you that you do need to exercise. It's essential that you find a form of exercise that you like. Play music that you love as you do it, as an extra motivation. Remember to tell your body that you love the exercise and soon enough it will love moving – whether through yoga, walking, trampolining or skipping, etc.

TURN DOWN THE HEATING

If your home, car and office are all heated your metabolic rate becomes slower. Turning down the heating and wearing a layer less boosts your metabolic rate as more calories are burned keeping you warm from the inside out. Sleeping in a very cool room makes your metabolic rate work harder throughout the night.

EAT LEAN PROTEIN

Eat fish, chicken, lentils, lean meat, nuts and eggs. Have some protein at every meal. The body works hard to properly digest protein so the longer and the more effort put into digesting protein, the more calories your body uses up and the more your metabolic rate will increase. Lean protein elevates metabolism by up to 10 per cent more than when carbs or fat are eaten.

CALCIUM

Calcium has fat-burning properties so a regular intake of calcium stimulates the mechanism in fat cells that break down fat. Get your calcium from soya foods, calcium-enriched rice milk, sheep's yogurt, broccoli, cauliflower, kale, sesame seeds, sunflower seeds, almonds and tahini paste.

POTASSIUM

Potassium-rich foods help to regulate both your metabolism and your body's water balance. Potassium is found in apricots, bananas, carrots, parsley, peas, spinach, salmon, sardines and cod.

JAPANESE GREEN TEA

This speeds up the metabolism because it contains chemicals called methylxanthines which seem to boost metabolism and burn fat more rapidly. If you don't like the taste you can buy it in capsule form.

SOYA MILK

Soy protein slightly increases your metabolism and seems to encourage weight loss from the middle. The isoflavones, glycine and arginine in soya milk seem to accelerate the breakdown of fat, reduce the levels of sugar in the blood and lower the level of insulin in the blood. You can consume your soya in soya flour, soya protein (tofu), soya yogurt, soya cheese and soy beans. *Not soy sauce*. Soya is also a very important anti-cancer food. Many people recognise it as a universal cancer preventative because the genestien and daidzien within it are anti-cancer agents.

HERBS

The herbs cinnamon, ginger, cayenne, cardamom and ginseng can help to stimulate thermogenesis (heat generated by the body) and promote weight loss.

SPICES

Hot spices can boost the rate at which calories are burned by up to 15 per cent for a few hours after eating. Chillies speed up the metabolism and reduce hunger. South Americans have known for years that chillies reduce appetite.

SUPPLEMENTS

Tyrosine-rich foods like pumpkin seeds, almonds and avocados feed the metabolism. Taking a tyrosine supplement (500mg four times daily) and a zinc supplement (50mg daily) will boost your levels of tyrosine and can help to stop compulsive eating. Iodine keeps the metabolism working properly, kelp supplements are full of iodine as are strawberries and seaweed.

Processed foods are full of additives and research shows that additives can interfere with the mechanisms involved in the metabolic process causing the metabolism to slow down. Check food labels for E-numbers to see how many additives the food contains.

FIDGET

I never thought I would promote fidgeting, I love calmness. However, those who fidget, twiddle pens, tap their feet up and down, rotate their feet around, or swing a crossed leg up and down or bounce their heels off the floor while queuing burn more calories than calm individuals. Nervy types burn off more nervous energy. NEAT = non-exercise-activity-thermogenesis, which is the name for continuous movement, can burn off 200 calories daily.

A New Kind of Takeaway With No Calories

By this stage in the book you have taken in so much information and implemented great changes with every exercise you have done, you are equipped with new habits for the new you. You have accomplished so much already and you can now move on and make the following actions – which are easy, convenient and inexpensive – a part of your daily life. Print them out and stick them on your fridge and remember they are designed to help you change your shape and size and *they work*.

1 Visualise yourself as thinner constantly.

2 Change your language and your beliefs, take control of how you talk, think, act and react with regard to food. Your mind begins to feed back to you the things you tell it, when you say 'I can cope if I eat biscuits' enough times your mind begins to remind you of this so stop giving your mind harmful beliefs.

Your body does not ask you to fill it with chemicals and sugar, it is your mind that does this and you can easily change this.

3 Use the three Rs to remind you to eat the food Mother Nature put on the planet for you:
Food that grows or *Roams*.
Food that you could eat *Raw*.
Food that you can *Recognise* as food.

4 Have your desk, office, locker, travel bag and car always stocked up with portable foods that you like and that sustain you so that you always have an alternative food handy.

5 Buy your food staples in bulk at least three at a time so that you don't run out of them. Shop online and have them delivered weekly if it makes it easier. Replace your portable foods and your pantry staples as soon as you use them.

6 Replace dairy foods with good substitutes.

7 Eat more slowly. Properly chewing food automatically makes us eat more slowly and we become full more quickly and hence eat less. Your nose is over your mouth for a reason, you are supposed to smell your food before you eat it, so slow down your eating pace and take the time to smell your food as well as taste it because smelling it tells the body how to digest it. Digestion begins in the mouth not the stomach the digestive enzymes in saliva are more powerful than those in our stomach.

8 Eat serotonin-producing foods every day to keep you happy and to beat cravings: coriander, bananas, eggs, avocados and turkey.

9 Put your own needs first and remember you are worth it. If

the foods you should be eating aren't available, ask your host or waiter for something different. In order to make someone else happy you have to take care of your own happiness first. Eat like celebrities who have no problem requesting special food because they know they are worth it, that they can get it by asking politely and that it is important to them. These are the same beliefs that allow people with allergies or religious needs to ask for different food.

10 Remember cereals are cattle feed and glue so they shouldn't be your primary food, and dairy is not suited to our bodies.

11 Stop eating starchy carbs after lunch.

12 Limit the variety of food at each meal.

13 Keep the right food in your house and the wrong food out of your house; especially don't buy it for others as it just leads to temptation.

14 Avoid fast food and any food with taste enhancers or additives.

15 Eat earlier and make late-night eating an exception not the rule.

So now you have takeaways that keep you thinner and you know what to do, the new thin you will never have to diet or go hungry again. You will eat better than you have eaten in the past but weigh less and feel happier. Like me you will wish that you had this information years ago as it will improve your relationship with food, with yourself and with everyone around you.

I am often very busy so I have to eat in this way. I spend a lot of time on the road travelling and spend weeks in different countries. I have had to devise a programme that encompasses the most difficult and challenging eating situations. Many diet books assume that the reader loves to cook and has time to cook. This is not always the case so many people turn to fast food because they don't have the time, the energy or the inclination to cook. Many of my clients frequently report that they are so hungry after a long day working that even while cooking for their family they end up snacking on junk like biscuits and bread perpetuating the negative eating cycle. Or they buy sandwiches and crisps and eat them on the way home not even bothering with a meal once they are home. Nowadays people buy more takeaways and more ready-cooked supermarket meals than ever before. So many families infrequently eat meals together and around the table and this has to be taken into account in any modern diet book.

If you love cooking and have time to cook healthy fresh food that is an asset. If you don't, you can still shed weight easily. This programme works for everyone from stressed-out mothers on a tight budget to executives. I work with lots of executives who live a five-star life and still eat the wrong things. Doing what I do will cut years of trial and error from your goal of being slimmer and add years to your life. It has taken me a long time and many years of studying my own clients to devise this method of becoming and remaining thinner with ease.

How to Shop and Feed Your Guests

When people come to your house for dinner or to stay as guests, give them the same type of food that you are now eating. You can adapt your new eating plan and, of course, you can buy cakes and pizza especially for your guests or your children and their friends if they are having a tea party or sleepover. Just make a point of buying desserts and biscuits that you don't like as it is so much easier to avoid them. If your least favourite crisps are salt and vinegar buy only those; if you hate biscuits with coconut or ginger in them buy those. If you are buying ice cream for a summer barbecue again buy the flavour that you don't like. I don't like rum and raisin ice cream so I can keep that in my house forever. If there are any leftovers encourage your guests to take them home when they leave or throw them away or put them in the freezer out of sight.

I am also very comfortable making my guests a pasta dinner if that is what they want while preparing something different for me and eating with them. The key is not to make a fuss and never to make a big deal about it. If you are relaxed and comfortable your guests will be the same. When I was a vegetarian I would cook meat for my daughter and sit with people eating meat and it was not an issue.

Avoid hosting or going out for afternoon tea because it is a time when only cakes and sandwiches are served. If you are invited to afternoon tea ask for a piece of fruit or take some with you. If you have to make afternoon tea include fruit and throw the biscuits away as soon as the guests have left.

When you are eating out ask for different food or for your food to be prepared differently without feeling embarrassed about it. Remember if you were diabetic you would do this because your health depended on it. Your health does depend on it too, so put your needs first politely and discreetly and no one else will care or probably even notice.

What to Eat

Your new way of eating for life involves eating primarily foods based around fruit, vegetables, salads, nuts, seeds, soya and lean protein. You can eat some complex carbohydrates like oats but not every day.

For breakfast you can have fruit with some almonds or soya yogurt with seeds, nuts and fruit, or a soya and fruit smoothie or scrambled eggs with coriander or oats with nuts or seeds made with water and soya or rice milk, or any kind of fish. Eat a banana daily as a snack and for lunch you can have protein, salad and vegetables and more fruit, for dinner you can have protein, salad and vegetables. You can add soups and sweet potatoes (as they are actually yams, not potatoes) to lunch and dinner, you can snack on fruit, seeds, nuts, edamame, smoothies and rice milk lattes. Your staple snack could be unsalted almonds – they are so good for us and so portable. In the winter you can make a lot more soups and in the summer snack much more on berries when they're in season and therefore cheaper. You can eat potatoes, rice, and bread but aim to not eat them daily and not after lunch. Quinoa is a much better choice than rice or potatoes to eat with meat or fish or put in soups and salads as it's a seed and a very healthy food that gives you a lot of energy.

You can have a varied healthy diet but limit the variety of food at each meal, for instance at breakfast you could have eggs or fish or oats with nuts and seeds and some fruit but don't have some of everything because this stimulates your appetite and encourages overeating. If you get hungry late at night try to have just fruit or hot tea as you cannot digest food late at night.

What to Visualise and Why

On the (occasional) days when you eat more than you need to you can easily visualise yourself burning it all off while you are sleeping. This is no different really to visualising yourself gaining weight except one is a positive visualisation the other is very negative. When you get offered sweets or a handful of someone else's crisps you can say, 'No I don't eat that stuff'. This isn't always true but say it all the time anyway as the more you say it the more true it becomes. The way we visualise is the way we become. You can become a walking talking affirmation of the way you want to be. Keep telling yourself you burn off food as a waking visualisation, too. And of course you are ready to play your audio download now. You can play it every day, more than once a day, as it will help you to visualise.

This is not an ending it's a new beginning. You have learned so much starting with changing your attitude and then your language before moving on to choosing to be thin. You have taken lots of small steps that get big results and you are finally able to get the body you want by making mental changes and welcoming some restrictions, because they bring results that make it worth it. You have learned to think thin and know that continuously visualising your body the way you want it to look is not some new age hocus pocus it is a science that really works. You know how to visualise your progress for lasting success and how to make brainwashing work for you not against you.

You have learned how to end cravings that are physical and mental and made changes from the inside as well as on the outside. As a grand finale you know how to keep it off forever and I know that you can do it. The Ten New Takeaways will help you keep on the straight and narrow and if you hit a curve you can just get right back on track. Don't ever give up just because you have eaten a biscuit, after all you wouldn't go on to empty out your bank account just because you have overspent would you? The definition of success is not if you fail but how quickly you get back on track if you do fail. A day in the life of the new thin you is how you are going to be almost all the time. The thing I love the most about my programme is that you don't have to do all of it all of the time for it to work. As long as you do most of it most of the time it will work.

It's essential that you have not only read this book from cover to cover but that you have done all the exercises required (if you have skipped any of them please go back and do them right now, not for me but for you). I designed these exercises so that you can be thin so please do them.

So what next? Be thinner, be happy and know that you are always enough. If you slip up go back to the appropriate chapter; if you are still hard on yourself reread the chapter on 'Changing Your Language'. If you still hanker after rubbish food reread 'How to End Cravings' and put the information into practice. If other people give you a hard time or try to make you eat the food that they like to eat reread 'How to Say No and Mean It'. And remember this is all about you, you don't need to convert anyone (unless of course they want you to in which case please do) and neither can anyone convert you back to those old bad habits unless you let them and you are never going to do that.

If any particular chapter in this programme really resonated with something inside you then go back and read that chapter again. Print out some of the sayings if they were particularly helpful and remember them.

Remember you have been through a hypnotic process and you have worked hard to make powerful and lasting changes. They won't undo themselves and if you are at all worried that they will remember you have an additional special tool, your audio download (see Contents page). Every time you play it you are reinforcing your mind and replacing old negative suggestions with powerful positive ones. As you play the audio download the image of you at your ideal weight will become more real and more attainable each time that you hear it. The audio download is going to help you so much. It will have a powerful, permanent and all-pervasive impact on your self image, your eating habits and your beliefs so play it every day without a break for twenty-one days (remember those neural pathways changing after twenty-one days) and then continue to play it regularly until the words become deeply embedded into your subconscious mind.

From start to finish of this book you have been absorbing powerful workable solutions to being overweight. You cannot adhere to this programme without feeling and seeing the benefits. As long as you use this book the way it was meant to be used you can be thin.

I hope you have enjoyed this journey to be thinner, to be cured of dieting forever. The destination is fantastic – it's you looking the way you were meant to look but the journey is quite an accomplishment too. Thank you so much for taking it with me. Please keep in touch with me and let me know your progress you can e mail me for advice on www.marisapeer.com or info@marisapeer.com

Here's looking at (the new thin) you.

Marisa Peer.

Afterword for the 2015 Edition

I have been telling my patients for years that sugar and low calorie starchy foods make us fat, whereas wonderful health-giving foods containing fat or protein keep us slim, and in the last few years I have noticed that finally nutritionists, doctors and scientists worldwide have come to the same conclusion. When I worked for Jane Fonda I lived on the LA diet of low calorie yogurt, diet coke, fruit, salad with no dressing and no fat and during that time, even though I was exercising a lot as one of Jane's trainers, I struggled every day to stay slim. Now I eat a very different diet – I eat eggs, fish, chicken, meat and vegetables, no more than three pieces of fruit daily and I snack on olives, avocados and nut butter on celery or sliced peppers. I never starve myself and I am slimmer than I ever was then.

It is quite simple. Protein is composed of amino acids that the body can't store, so when you eat protein your body uses it as a building food to repair your body and is quickly used and not stored as fat. When you eat carbohydrates they are stored as fat unless you burn them off with a lot of exercise. That is why body builders only eat protein and vegetables before competitions because they want to stay in fat-burning mode so their muscles are more visible. Carbs, on the other hand, are designed to give you energy. If you eat carbs and then do activities like exercise or hard manual work they get burnt off, but if you eat them and stay sedentary – i.e. at your desk – then instead of using carbs your body stores the excess as energy as fat.

When you eat carbs or any starchy food they turn to sugar very fast (grains are 70–80 per cent starch) and when your blood sugar goes up you make insulin, the job of which is for fat storage. It's harder to lose weight once you have eaten carbs and it's harder to gain weight without eating carbs.

You have a 90 per cent chance of remaining overweight if your diet is high in carbohydrates and starchy foods. The reason for this is that to burn fat you have to reduce sugar but your body cannot differentiate between carbs and sugar, they are equally recognised and both used by your body as sugar. Once you have eaten the equivalent of three teaspoons of sugar you are now in fat-storing mode and if you eat starch three or four times a day you are constantly making your body store fat and never giving it the opportunity to burn off. Eating pasta, rice, potatoes and bread is no different to eating cake and as you recognise this it becomes easier to adapt your eating to allow your body to burn fat. You would not eat cake at every meal so seeing starchy carbs as no different to cake makes it easier to limit them.

Your body reacts differently to calories composed of fat and protein than it does to calories composed of carbohydrates. Only carbohydrates stimulate your pancreas to release insulin and the job of insulin is to store fat. Every single time you eat carbs they become glucose (sugar) which is only ever any kind of benefit if you need that glucose to burn as energy. If you have no need for the energy because you are sedentary (or because you already have a lot of energy stored as surplus fat) your body will store further excess energy as more fat and for many of us this happens several times a day, every day. That is why shifting the excess weight is hard, we never get to use up our fat deposits and we keep making more of them simply because when we have glucose in our body we cannot use up any of our existing stored fat. However without glucose (carbs) in our body our insulin levels drop and we switch to fat burning rather than fat storing.

When carbohydrates are restricted fat is broken down and when you eat more carbs than your body can use the excess is converted to fat. Your body simply cannot burn fat and shed weight when you eat carbs several times a day because it never gets the chance to burn off the fat that you keep storing at every meal and snack. That three teaspoons of sugar that I mentioned is not a lot at all, once you have consumed that amount your body is at full carb capacity and any more will be stored as fat. When you restrict carbs you always burn fat and shed weight so when you wake up in the morning you are at peak fat-burning capacity and you will stay that way until you next eat a carb. If you remind yourself of this you are more motivated to breakfast on eggs with green vegetables knowing that by doing this you will stay in fat-burning mode until your next meal. This may motivate you to ensure your next meal is carb free too and, although you don't have to do this all the time, just doing this a few times a week will make your body more adept at burning fat and losing weight.

Switching carbs for protein or carbs for fat helps you train your body to burn fat. This means switching crisps or crackers for nuts or olives. Swap granola or cereal bars for celery or pepper slices spread with crunchy nut butter. Replace rice and pasta with quinoa or amaranth or julienned courgettes. In place of potatoes roast Jeruselam artichokes or dry roast cauliflower florets.

When you eat protein you burn fat; when you eat carbs you store fat. But when you add protein to carbs you slow down the sugar. This means that if you really want a pasta or rice dish add a protein like fish or chicken to make it less starchy. A better way to monitor your diet is to never double carb. This simply means that if you have a baked potato, don't add baked beans or you will be eating two types of starchy carbs together. Instead add tuna or a poached egg. When eating toast instead of adding jam or honey have natural almond nut butter or a slice of ham so you are slowing the sugar down rather than increasing it. Eat ryvita with nut butter or avocado rather than honey and if you want oats for breakfast add a few nuts and seeds and use nut milk like almond milk to slow down the sugar. Adding banana, raisins and honey to oats makes it ultra-high in sugar. Don't have tomato based sauces with rice or pasta; add fish or lean meat so you eat one carb and one protein instead of two carbs. Eating two carbs together is giving your body twice the sugar and twice the amount of fat storage.

Get into the habit of asking yourself two questions just before you eat as this will help you to make better choices. Ask yourself 'will my body store this as fat or use it, is this food fat burning or fat storing?' and 'where is the protein?'

If you have a three egg omelette stuffed with vegetables you will burn it off and stay full for hours, whereas if you have cereal and milk or toast and jam your body can't use up the high amount of carbs and must instead store the excess as fat. However, if you have toast and add an egg or a slice of ham instead of jam the protein slows down the sugar and you stay the same – neither burning or storing fat. When I am eating out – especially if it's a Sunday lunch – I refuse potatoes and order twice as many veg and have extra protein as the mistake so many people make is to refuse the carbs and end up with a piece of chicken or fish and a few vegetables which are not enough. You must eat more protein and more vegetables so you feel you have eaten enough. I know that taking away potatoes or Yorkshire pudding will keep me in fat-burning mode whereas adding them to my meal takes me out of it, and although I don't do this all the time I do it enough of the time to stay slim.

When you live on a low fat diet you will just end up craving fat and then binge on of crisps and chocolate, so instead eat good fats regularly and when you crave sugar eat a big spoon of nut butter instead or half an avocado or some olives or unsalted nuts – this really works to stop the craving. My favourite snack is to slice an apple or a red pepper and spread the slices with any kind of nut butter like almond butter or peanut butter this quickly ends a sugar craving.

Just remember that the key to making your body a fantastic fat-burning machine is to avoid or lessen starchy carbohydrates because your body is designed to store carbohydrates as energy and if you don't burn off that energy it will always be stored as fat. Limiting when and how you eat them is the key to permanent weight loss. I love fruit but I restrict myself to three pieces a day most of the time. Vegetables are far more important than fruits they have more vitamins and antioxidants and we should have more daily servings of vegetables than fruit. Fruit is still a sugar and too much of it pushes up insulin levels. Fruit juice is not a good food at all as it contains way too much sugar.

I have included some recipes and meal ideas for you. Please remember that this is for you to adapt in a way that suits you and works for you so that you can make it a way of life.

RECIPES

Three eggs – either scrambled with olive or coconut oil, or a three egg omelette cooked in oil. Remember: no milk or butter. Add mushrooms, herbs, spinach, peppers, leeks, onions or any green veg for flavour and variety. You can also add a little real ham, bacon or smoked salmon or prawns.

Soya yogurt with a 10–15 almonds or a dessert spoonful of seeds either sunflower, hemp, sesame or pumpkin or any mixed seeds and nuts, add a teaspoon of cinnamon as it speeds up your metabolism.

Bacon, or turkey bacon, and eggs with spinach or mushrooms.

MORNING AND AFTERNOON SNACKS

Soya yogurt with a small handful of seeds or nuts
Edemame beans with a little light soya sauce
20oz hummus with raw vegetables like celery and peppers
Handful of raw nuts
Green apple, pear or berries

CHICKEN SALAD

Serves 4

For the Dressing:
$1/2$ cup olive oil
$1/4$ cup balsamic vinegar
$1/8$ teaspoon coriander

Salad Ingredients:
2 cups cooked chicken, cut into cubes
Tomatoes,
Peppers
Cucumber
Spring onions

In a small bowl, combine the olive oil, vinegar, and coriander.

In a medium bowl, place all the remaining ingredients. Whip the dressing ingredients together with a fork, and then pour over the chicken mixture.

Gently toss and refrigerate until served.

TERIYAKI TURKEY

Serves 4

1¹/4 pounds turkey pieces (this can also be substituted for beef)
5 tablespoons teriyaki sauce, divided
2 tablespoons sugar-free peanut butter
¹/4 teaspoon ground ginger
1 tablespoon (or more to taste) low sugar or sugar-free Hot Chili
   Sauce
2 tablespoons vegetable oil
¹/2 cup cucumber, seeded and chopped

Cut turkey into ¹/8 inch thick strips.

In medium bowl, combine turkey and 2 tablespoons teriyaki
sauce; toss to coat.

In small bowl, combine remaining 3 tablespoons teriyaki sauce,
peanut butter, 1 tablespoon water, ginger and hot chili sauce.

Meanwhile, in large nonstick pan or wok, heat oil over
medium-high heat until hot. Add turkey (¹/2 at a time) and stir-fry
for 1 to 2 minutes or until outside surface is no longer pink.

Remove turkey from wok. Toss turkey with peanut butter mixture to coat.

Sprinkle with chopped cucumber.

Serves 4

2 teaspoons finely minced garlic
1 cup chopped onions
1 large aubergine
3 medium courgettes
2 large green peppers
1 teaspoon dried oregano
1 tablespoon fresh basil or 2 teaspoons dried basil
2 teaspoons chopped parsley
2 cups crushed canned tomatoes
Fresh ground pepper

Cut vegetables into 1-inch pieces.

Heat oil in large pan and add the garlic and onions. Cook until tender.

Add the aubergine, courgette, pepper, oregano, parsley and stir well – sauté for about 5 minutes.

Add tomatoes, cover and cook over low heat for about 45 minutes.

Serve hot or cover mixture and refrigerate to serve chilled.

GARLIC-GINGER CHICKEN STRIPS

Serves 2

2 skinless boneless chicken breast halves
$1/4$ cup soy sauce
1 tablespoon fresh basil
6 to 8 cloves garlic, minced
2 teaspoons grated ginger root
$1/2$ pepper
$1/2$ teaspoon crushed red pepper
$1/2$ teaspoon five-spice powder

Cut each chicken breast half lengthwise into 4 long strips.

In a medium non-metal bowl, combine all other ingredients. Mix well.

Add chicken pieces and cover with marinade. Let marinate for 15 minutes at room temperature or 4–24 hours refrigerated.

Drain chicken. Place chicken pieces on hot grill, grill 4–5 inches from heat about 5 minutes or until light brown. Turn and grill another 3–5 minutes until golden brown and no longer pink inside.

Serve hot with mixed roast vegetables such as peppers, onions. leeks, courgettes and tomatoes.

Serves 1

2 teaspoon oil
1 garlic clove, crushed
1 spring onion, finely chopped
2 teaspoons finely chopped fresh root ginger
1 green chilli, deseeded and finely chopped
Juice from $1/2$ lime
100g raw prawns, any size
165ml can coconut milk
100ml chicken or vegetable stock
2 courgettes julienned
Chopped coriander, to serve

Heat the oil in a large pan or wok. When hot, add the garlic, spring onion, ginger and green chilli. Cook on a medium heat for 3–4 mins, then squeeze in lime juice.

Stir in the prawns, then add in the coconut milk and stock. Simmer gently for 5 mins on a low heat until the prawns are pink.

Meanwhile, boil or fry the julienned courgette noodles for 1–2 minutes.

Drain, then tip into the laksa pan. Season to taste and serve in a bowl, topped with coriander.

CHUNKY FISHCAKES

Serves 2

4 portions of fish either salmon, tuna, cod or haddock (about
    400g) either fresh, frozen or canned chopped into bite size
    chunks
2 tablespoons of red or green thai curry paste
1oz grated ginger
1 large bunch of fresh coriander roughly shredded
1 teaspoon olive or sunflower oil
1 teaspoon light soya sauce

Mix the fish in a food processor with the paste, ginger, soya sauce
and coriander until roughly blended.

Remove mix and form into 4 round or oblong fish cakes.

Heat the oil in wok or frying pan and fry the burgers for 4–5
minutes on each side, turning until crisp and cooked through.
You can also fry them in pure lemon juice and no oil or use spray
oil.

Serve with julienned courgettes, stir-fried Savoy cabbage or
roasted peppers and red onions.

FAVA BEAN FALAFEL

1 tin fava beans, drained, or 1 cup of dried peeled fava beans
   soaked overnight with half a cup of soaked or drained chickpeas
1 chopped red onion or three chopped scallions
2 cloves of garlic, chopped
2 tablespoons of fresh parsley, chopped
Medium size bunch of fresh coriander chopped
1 teaspoon cumin
$1/2$ teaspoon baking powder
Salt and pepper
2 tablespoons olive oil for baking

Make sure the ingredients are dry rather than wet then place the
beans in a blender and blend.

Add the rest of the ingredients apart from the oil and blend
again to form a smooth but thick paste, if too thick add 1 tablespoon of water at a time until it is the correct consistency.

Form the mixture into small balls or patties.

Arrange on a tray and leave to stand in the fridge for 30 minutes.

Drizzle the oil evenly into a baking dish and preheat oven to
180. Place the mixture into the baking dish and oven bake for
15–20 minutes turning halfway through cooking. Serve with vegetables or salad drizzled with tahini sauce.

Make extra to take with you for lunch they are just as delicious
cold.

Soups

SPICY TOMATO SOUP

Makes 6 servings

8 fresh tomatoes pureed
1 cup of water
1 cup of chicken broth
1 red onion finely minced
2 gloves of garlic mixed
2 red peppers diced
1 teaspoon of cayenne pepper
1 teaspoon paprika
1/4 green chillies diced
1/4 chives diced

Combine all ingredients in a large soup pot and cook on low heat for one hour.

Makes 6 servings

6 cups of water
Meat of 1 chicken diced
2 cloves of garlic diced
2 onions diced
1 teaspoon black pepper
18 button mushrooms

In a large pan combine water chicken, garlic, onion, bay leaf and pepper.

Bring to boil then reduce heat cover and simmer for 2 hours until chicken is tender.

Remove bay leaf and bring to boil again.

Reduce heat and add mushrooms. Cover, then simmer for 20 minutes.

CABBAGE SOUP

Makes 6–8 servings

3 cups non-fat broth (beef, chicken or vegetable)
2 garlic cloves, minced
1 tablespoon tomato paste
2 cups chopped cabbage
$1/2$ yellow onion
$1/2$ cup chopped carrots
$1/2$ cup green beans
$1/2$ cup chopped courgette
$1/2$ teaspoon basil
$1/2$ teaspoon oregano
Salt & pepper to taste

In a large saucepan sprayed with non-stick cooking spray, sauté carrot, onion and garlic over low heat for 5 minutes (until softened).

Add broth, tomato paste, cabbage, green beans, basil, oregano, and salt & pepper to taste.

Lower heat and simmer for about 10–15 minutes until all vegetables are tender.

Stir in courgette and heat 3–4 minutes. Serve hot.

ALTERNATIVE TO SPAGHETTI

Julienne courgettes by slicing them lengthways with a julienne or a potato peeler if you don't have one (they are so cheap and worth getting). Once you have a mound of spaghetti-looking courgette ribbons place them in pan of boiling water for just one minute then drain well and add to meatballs, meat sauces or any other dish where you previously would have used pasta. You can also stir fry them in oil for just two minutes.

ALTERNATIVE TO RICE

Take a head of cauliflower cut into chunks and discard the core as it's too bitter while keeping the florets. Add the florets to a food processor and use the grating blade to grate until the whole cauliflower has been used. The cauliflower crumbles really fast so give it a blast of a few seconds then check it out and repeat until its all crumbled. Once you have your mound of rice you can add it to salads, curries and sauces raw or any dish that would have previously used rice. Or you can cook it for no more than a minute with a little oil in a wok and then add ingredients to it or use it as the base for dishes like Spanish Rice, Savoury Rice, Rissotto, Kedgeree (my favourite). You can also used cooked mashed cauliflower as a great topping for shepherd's pie or fish pie.

ALTERNATIVE POTATOES

Roast Jerusalem artichokes taste very similar to roast potatoes. If you are making a shepherd's pie you can make the topping with mashed cauliflower. Mashed cauliflower or mashed carrot and swede are a great substitute for mashed potato.

Cook a large pan of porridge oats using water or water and rice, oat or soya milk.

Once it is cooked through leave it to absorb all the liquid and thicken then add other ingredients to it like hemp seeds and microwaved popcorn, or sunflower seeds, flaked almonds, sesame seeds, pumpkin seeds.

Pour the mixture onto a baking tray and cook in the oven for about 20 minutes. If you like it chewy cook it for less time and if you like it crunchy press it down so it is thinner and cook for a little longer then cut into squares or slices and enjoy.

You can experiment with lots of added ingredients like chopped up pear and ginger or grated apple and cinnamon or mashed up banana and peanut butter (smooth or crunchy and of course sugar free) or blueberries or any berries and desiccated coconut. In fact any kind of fruit, seeds, nut combo is good; don't use dried any fruit as it is too high in sugar.

These bars will keep for at least a week in foil or an airtight container and are great for breakfast on the go, or as alternatives to biscuits and snacks for adults and children.

400g tinned chickpeas drained
2 tablespoons light tahini paste
2 crushed garlic cloves
Juice of 1 lemon (you can also add lime juice)
2-5 tablespoons virgin olive oil
Small handful of parsley
Small handful of coriander
Half teaspoon mild smoked paprika
2–4 tablespoons water according to how thick you like it

Blend all the ingredients in a food processor season with salt and or black pepper.

Spoon into a tub or individual bowls and place in fridge for an hour before serving. It will thicken up so you can thin it with more water or olive oil.

Sprinkle with smoked paprika or tumeric for colour and a few sprigs of corinader or parsley.

You can make hummus different by adding tomatoes, peppers, olives or sun dried tomatoes to the mix. If you have time it's lovely to roast or grill peppers or tomatoes or a mild red chilli or all three for about 7 minutes until the skins blacken then remove the skins and add the roasted peppers, chilli and or tomatoes to the mix before blending.

When you add ingredients like cucumber, tomatoes or peppers you naturally lower the calories, just make sure the salad ingredients have been dried in kitchen towels so they don't make the hummus watery.

KALE CRISPS

Take 12 large kale leaves (wash, rub, dry, and cut in half lengthwise, taking care to remove the stem and veins)
1–2 tablespoons of olive or sesame oil

Preheat oven to 140 °C.

Toss kale leaves in a large bowl with the oil so they are coated.

Sprinkle with salt and pepper and lemon juice (optional). If you
like a bit of spice, you can also add a tea spoon of chili flakes.
Garlic flakes or toasted garlic sprinkled on top works well too.

Arrange leaves in a single layer on 2 large baking trays.

Bake until crisp, about 25 minutes for flat leaves and up to 30
minutes for wrinkled leaves. Allow to cool.

You can cut the kale into bite size pieces but they look impressive in halves and are great for dips.

One cup peanut butter (crunchy or smooth)
Three table spoons xylitol (tastes and bakes just like sugar)
1 large egg
Shredded coconut (optional – gives more texture)

Simply whisk ingredients together in a bowl and place on cookie sheet.

Bake for about 10–12 minutes at 200 °C, or until firm.

Let cookies sit for 5 minutes or so after baking as the texture will change and they will firm up a bit.

LOW CARB FAT-BURNING PANCAKES

Makes 6–8 pancakes

8 egg whites
2–4 egg yolks
50–60g of almond flour
Coconut oil for frying

Blend all ingredients together using either hand blender or food processor until it forms a thick consistency.

Heat a frying pan over a medium heat and add the coconut oil.

Once the oil is hot, add a ladle of the batter. Wait until the pancake starts to bubble on the top then turn it over. Cook both sides until they are brown.

Repeat until you have used up all the batter.

SERVE WITH:

Berries
Coyo yogurt
Any nut or seed butter
Lemon juice

125ml almond milk
2 tablespoons ground flaxseed or linseed
285g sieved spelt flour
75g unsweetened cocoa powder (preferably raw)
1¹/₄ teaspoons bicarbonate of soda
175g chocolate chips
125ml sunflower oil
190g natural granulated Xylitol
1 tablespoon vanilla extract

Preheat oven to 180 °C & grease 2 baking sheets

Mix the almond milk with the ground flaxseed or linseed, set aside to thicken.

Separately, mix the sieved flour, cocoa powder, and bicarbonate of soda in a large bowl and stir in chocolate chips.

Add the sunflower oil, sweetener and vanilla to the milk-seed mixture and stir thoroughly.

Leave for 5 minutes to thicken again then pour it into the bowl of dry ingredients and stir to combine. Set aside for 10–15 minutes to firm up.

Pinch off walnut sized pieces, roll them into balls in your palms, then flatten into discs about 1cm thick.

Arrange on baking sheets with space to spread.

Bake in the preheated oven for about 7 minutes. Let them cool slightly and harden on the sheets and then transfer to a wire rack to cool.

HEMP SEED MUFFINS WITH ORANGE

125g quinoa flower
$^1/_2$ teaspoon bicarbonate of soda
1 teaspoon baking powder
$^1/_2$ teaspoon salt
1 teaspoon ground cardamom
1 teaspoon ground cinnamon
2–3 heaped tablespoons shelled hemp seeds
1 teaspoon orange oil (or orange extract
1 tablespoon apple cider vinegar
100ml unsweetened apple puree
60ml almond milk
2 teaspoons xylitol

Preheat oven to 180 °C and line mini muffin pan with baking cups

In a bowl, combine quinoa flower, bicarbonate of soda, baking powder, and salt, then sift in spices. Add hemp seeds.
In separate bowl mix orange oil, apple puree, milk, and xylitol.
Mix the wet ingredients into the bowl of dry (don't over mix).
Spoon mixture into muffin cases filling them three-quarters.
Bake in oven for 10–12 minutes (a bit less if you like them moist on the inside).
Allow to cool before serving.

$1^1/_2$ tablespoons ground flaxseed
$4^1/_2$ tablespoons water
150g gluten free plain flour
2 teaspoons baking powder
1 teaspoon bicarbonate of soda
$^3/_4$ teaspoon salt
2 teaspoons ground cinnamon
$^1/_2$ teaspoons ground ginger
190g xylitol
125ml apple puree
60ml almond milk
125ml olive oil
190g finely grated carrots
Handful of raisins
Handful of walnuts

Preheat oven to 180 °C and grease a cake tin with olive oil

Put the flaxseeds/linseeds and water in a small bowl and whisk until it is the consistency of a beaten egg; place in fridge.

In a larger bowl combine flour, baking powder, bicarbonate of soda, salt, cinnamon, ginger and nutmeg.

In a separate bowl, mix together xylitol, apple puree, almond milk and olive oil. Stir in water and seed mix, then pour entire mixture into dry ingredients and stir until smooth. Add carrots and raisins until they are evenly distributed.

Spoon the mixture into your cake tin and scatter walnuts on top. Bake in over for about 30 minutes, then cover will foil and return to oven for another 10-15 minutes.

Allow to cool thoroughly.

CHOCOLATE BERRY MOUSSE

1 cup frozen berries
1 ripe avocado
1¹/₂ cup baby spinach leaves
6 tablespoons cocoa powder (no need for this to be sweetened)
1 teaspoon xylitol (you don't need any more as the berries are sweet enough)
Pinch vanilla extract
2 small handfuls of ice

Blend all ingredients using a food processor or blender. Garnish with mint or berries and serve immediately.

2 teaspoons chia seeds (you can buy these ready-ground or simply
    put them in a coffee grinder)
2 tablespoons water
170g of ground almonds (or almond flour)
3 tablespoons unsweetened desiccated coconut
1 teaspoon ground cinnamon
$1/2$ teaspoon ground nutmeg
1 teaspoon baking powder
pinch of salt
few drops of vanilla extract
3 teaspoons xylitol
2 tablespoons almond milk

Preheat oven to 180 °C and line a baking sheet with parchment
paper

Combine chia seeds and water in a small bowl. Whisk together
until the mixture is the consistency of a beaten egg.

Combine 1 cup almond flour and combine with coconut, cinnamon, nutmeg, baking powder and salt.

Add the chia mixture, vanilla, xylitol and almond milk to the
bowl of dry ingredients and mix.

Divide mixture and shape into bite-sized balls (around 15) and
then flatten with palms to make cookies.

Arrange on baking sheet.

Bake in oven for 6 minutes, transfer to wire rack to cool
completely.

Notes

p. 7 'Change the feelings ...': Gil Boyne, *The Rules of the Mind*, www.gil-boyneonline.com

p. 20 'rules of the mind ...': ibid

p. 34 'goal-seeking creatures ...': Brian Tracy, *Psychology of Achievement* (Illinois, Nightingale Conant), 1994. Brian Tracy, *Goals!* (San Francisco, Berrett-Koehher), 2003

p. 37 'while doing research ...': Great Ormond Street Hospital, study in the effects of refined carbohydrates on epilepsy, www.gosh.nhs.uk/medical-information/procedures-and treatments/ketogenic-diet/

p. 43 'polycystic ovary syndrome ...': Polycystic ovary syndrome is a health problem that can affect a woman's menstrual cycle and fertility. Researchers believe insulin is linked to PCOS. For many women with PCOS, their bodies have problems using insulin so that too much remains in the body. Many women with PCOS are overweight. Eating less processed and sugary foods lowers blood sugar and improves the body's use of insulin and can normalise hormone levels. Even a 10 per cent reduction in body weight can restore a woman's period. www.womenshealth.gov, p.1. Women who are overweight can suffer from PCOS because their cells are resistant to insulin. This insulin resistance prevents cells using sugar in the blood normally and sugar is stored as fat instead. Dr David Cohill, gynaecologist

p. 46 'unleashes free radicals ...': Free radicals are a naturally occurring process in our bodies whereby atoms or groups or atoms lose their stable properties, split and lose an electron. They then try to stabilise by attaching to the nearest stable molecule and attempting to steal one of its electrons. The cascading effect of this damages and destroys cells and accelerates ageing. Being overweight unleashes more free radicals.

p. 47 'risk of strokes ...': Fat stored around the stomach near organs causes more insulin resistance. www.diabetes.org, *Diabetes Forecast*, February 2004.

Fat stored around the middle linked to high blood pressure, diabetes and heart disease. Neal Barnard, MD, *Vegetarian Times*, July/August 2005. Visceral fat (known as stomach or belly fat) is more dangerous than subcutaneous fat. Subcutaneous fat accounts for most of our flab/excess fat. Visceral fat is located at deeper levels and a surplus of deep fat in the abdomen effects major organs. The hormones released by visceral fat can inflame organs and can cause thrombosis. Visceral fat seems to have a bad effect on the way cells work with insulin. www.diabetes.org.

p. 51 'definitions of madness ...': Dr David Viscott, *The Making of a Psychiatrist* (London, Allison & Busby), 1973

p. 61 'a subconscious self . . .': Émile Coué (French pharmacist and psychologist, 1857–1926), *Self Mastery Through Conscious Autosuggestion* (London, Allen & Unwin), 1922.
Martin L. Rossman, *Guided Imagery for Self-healing* (California, New World Library), 2000

p. 61 'willpower and imagination . . .': Émile Coué, *Self Mastery Through Conscious Autosuggestion*

p. 61 'imagination is far more . . .': Gil Boyne, *The Rules of the Mind*

p. 62 'the way you think . . .': Martin L. Rossman, MD. Vivid imagery can send a message from the cerebral cortex to the lower brain centres, including the limbic system, the emotional centre of the brain. From there, the message is relayed to the endocrine system and the autonomic nervous system, which can affect a range of bodily functions. Martin L. Rossman, *Guided Imagery for Self-healing*.

p. 65 'visualisation skills significantly . . .': Dr Herbert Beason, Harvard University.
Newsweek, 'Mind, Body, Medicine' programme, 27 September 2004.
Dr Alan Logan, ND, FRSH, www.drlogan.com.
Bernie Sigel and Barbara Hoberman Levine, *Your Body Believes Every Word You Say* (Connecticut, Wordswork Press), 2000.

p. 66 'neurological habit pathways . . .': Stanford Brain Research Institute, Stanford University School of Medicine, http://med.stanford.edu.

p. 103 'biggest factors in . . .': Dr David Viscott, *The Making of a Psychiatrist*.

p. 103 'the happy hormone . . .': Massachusetts Institute of Technology, studies in serotonin by Dr Judith Wurtman, author of *Managing Your Mind Through Food* (London, HarperCollins), 1988.

p. 103 'bulimics, compulsive eaters . . .': ibid.

p. 104 'high carbohydrate diet . . .': *The Journal of Nutritional and Environmental Medicine* (London, Taylor & Francis)
Eric Schlosser, *Fast Food Nation* (London, Houghton Mifflin), 2001.

p. 105 'lack of dopamine . . .': Dopamine is a neurotransmitter involved in the neural circuits controlling appetite and pleasure and therefore plays a role in imbalances that result in disorders such as addiction and depression.

p. 105 'serotonin is made from . . .': Tryptophan is the amino acid that the body uses to make serotonin. Foods high in B vitamins like bananas and avocados convert the amino acid tryptophan into serotonin. So by eating these you are naturally helping your body produce more serotonin. *The American Journal of Clinical Nutrition* (Texas, The American Society for Nutrition), October 1985, p.639-643.

p. 106 'sunlight also helps . . .': Serotonin levels increase when we are exposed to bright sunlight. SSRIs (like Prozac) work by helping naturally produced serotonin stay in the bloodstream longer, keeping our mood and energy levels higher. Sunlight does this naturally – a major reason why moods tend to be elevated in the summer. www.cnn.com, 'Summer Sun for Winter Blues', July 1990.

p. 106 'an artificial sweetener . . .': David Steinman, *Diet for a Poisoned Planet* (London, Crown), 1990.

p. 107 'several new studies . . .': Medical Research Council, Human Nutrition Research Laboratory, Cambridge. http://www.lib.cam.ac.uk.

p. 107 'research has found . . .': Research by Judith Rapaport for the National Institute of Health Research at Oxford Brookes University, c.1980. http://www.nih.gov/.

p. 108 'obese pregnant women . . .': Dr Gary Shaw, University of California, Birth Defects Monitoring Programme, December 1999.

p. 109 'eliminating refined carbs . . .': Trans fats are fats that are artificially created through a chemical process of the hydrogenation of oil that solidifies the oil. They are considered harmful to our health.
Insulin resistance is a condition whereby the cells of the body become resistant to the effects of insulin. To compensate, more insulin is secreted when glucose builds up in the blood. It can lead to Type 2 diabetes.

p. 109 'In an experiment . . .': Great Ormond Street Hospital, www.gosh.nhs.uk

p. 109 'Researchers are beginning . . .': Dr Neil Ward, chemistry department, University of Surrey
CM Carter et al., 'Effects of a few foods diet in attention deficit disorder' (London, *Archives of Disease in Childhood*), 1993

p. 112 'Sugar creates an . . .': Natural Nutrition, http://www.livrite.com/.
William Duffy, *Sugar Blues* (New York, Grand Central Publishing), 1986.

p. 117 'consuming any dairy . . .': Dairy scientists have admitted that the level of a very powerful hormone contained in milk, insulin-like growth factor-I (IGF-I), increases in the human body after milk consumption. In the last two years, IGF-I has been identified as the key factor in the growth and proliferation of various cancers including prostate cancer and breast cancer. Many experts believe that the IGF-I in milk and lactose (a type of milk sugar found in milk) may over-stimulate hormones which may encourage tumour growth. The higher our levels of IGF, the higher our risk of developing certain cancers. Researchers at Stanford University and the National Institutes of Health found that high concentrations of the IGF-1 hormone stimulate cancer cell growth.
The Journal of the National Cancer Institute, vol. 91, no. 2, January 1999. *The Lancet*, vol. 351, May 1998. *Science*, vol. 279, January 1998.

p. 117 'When adult humans . . .': Milk is a concentrated source of chemical messengers, each one with a mission to influence the growth of a newborn.
Dr Jane Plant, *Your Life in Your Hands* (London, Virgin Books), 2006

p. 118 'can be disruptive . . .': University of Illinois scientist Dr Samuel Epstein warns that elevated levels of IGF-1 in milk from cows injected with rBGH is a potential risk factor for breast cancer in humans who consume cow's milk. IGF-1 is increasingly abundant in milk from cows treated with synthetic bovine growth hormone (rBGH). *International Journal of Health Sciences*
Dr Jane Plant, *Your Life in Your Hands*

p. 118 'Some researchers believe . . .': The Harvard Medical School's Guide to Healthy Eating (2001)
Harvard Nurses' Health Study

International renowned nutrition expert Dr. T. Colin Campbell

Dr Neal Barnard president of the Physicians Committee for Responsible Medicine

David Steinman

p. 118 'the machines extract . . .': www.dumpdairy.com

p. 118 '50 per cent mucus . . .': 1 teaspoon of milk can contain 2 million pus cells. In the EU milk is allowed to be sold when it contains 400,000 somatic pus cells per ml. The United States Department of Agriculture (USDA) does not allow milk containing 750 million or more pus cells per litre to cross state borders. EU directive 92/46/EEC.

p. 118 'Even pregnant cows . . .': The milk of pregnant cows contains pregnancy hormones including growth hormones, female sex hormones oestrogen and progesterone, and DHT. Harvard School of Public Health, *Journal of American Academy and Dermatology*.

p. 119 'Cheese protein has . . .': Studies published in the *Journal of the American Dietetic Association* and the *British Medical Journal*

p. 119 'Asians who consume . . .': T. Colin Cambell, 'The China Study'

p. 120 'The Masaii are . . .': www.notmilk.com African people experience little or no episodes of osteoporosis. The one exception is the milk-drinking Masaii.

p. 120 'No human can . . .': Lactase is an enzyme in young children, it is essential for digesting the lactose in milk. Deficiency of the enzyme lactase causes lactose intolerance (http://en.wikipedia.org/wiki/Lactose_intolerance). The journal of the American Dietetic Association reported in 1996 that 75 per cent of the world's population is lactose intolerant

p. 127 'milk containing 750 million . . .': EU directive 92/46/EEC.

p. 130 'introduction of grains . . .': *The Journal of Nutritional and Environmental Medicine* (London, Taylor & Francis)

p. 131 'Primitive man could not . . .': Most cereals are virtually indigestible unless the cell wall is broken down by milling and cooking.

p. 134 'fat stored around . . .': A study published in the Lancet in August 2004 led by Dr David Ludwig of The Children's Hospital, Boston

p. 134 'unnatural amount of gas . . .': A natural amount of gas is passing gas 14 to 24 times a day.

p. 137 'over 70 per cent . . .': Per cent of overweight adults in the Western world by country:
74% of Americans, 68.4% of New Zealanders, 68.1% of Mexicans, 67% of Australians, 66% of Canadians, 66% of Britons and 60% of Germans. These are the statistics for adults – when you factor in children and teenagers the figures are higher than 70%. www.forbes.com.

p. 138 'impairment of the . . .': Dr Arthur Agatston, *The South Beach Diet* (London, Headline), 2003

p. 151 'Eating fast food . . .': Morgan Spurlock, *Don't Eat This Book: Fast Food and the Supersizing of America* (London, Putnam), 2005

p. 152 'suggests fat and sugar . . .': Morgan Spurlock, *Don't Eat This Book: Fast Food and the Supersizing of America*

p. 153 'can be as dangerous . . .': Fatty liver means more fat in the liver than normal and is caused by obesity. Excessive fat in the diet can accumulate in the liver.

p. 153 'risk of diabetes ...': *The Lancet*, Fast food habits, weight gain and insulin, January 2005.

Stanford University School of Mecicine research.

Dr David Ludwig, Director of the Obesity Programme, Children's Hopital, Boston.

http://www.newstarget.com/.

p. 161 'eggs are a wonder food ...': The British Egg Information Service (BEIS), http://www.britegg.co.uk/.

The British Egg Industry Council (BEIC), www.britisheggindustrycouncil.co.uk/

p. 168 'boost metabolism and burn fat ...': *The American Journal of Clinical Nutrition* showed that green tea rich in catechins (natural plant chemicals) can reduce waist circumference and abdominal fat. The catechins can boost metabolism and burn fat.

To find out more information on Marisa and her books go to:

www.marisapeer.com

To get in contact you can email or call Marisa's office using the details below:

info@marisapeer.com
0207 736 4370

Or via social media:

www.facebook.com/marisa.peer.therapy

@marisapeer

www.marisapeer.blogspot.com